FANTASTIC

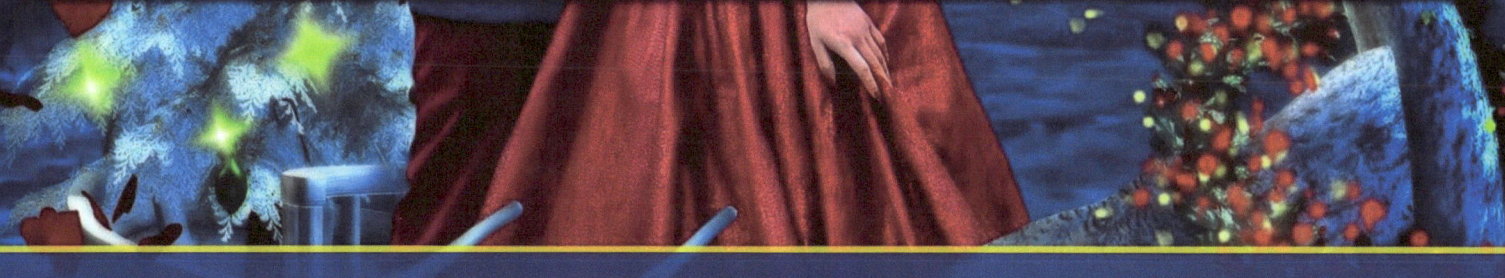

PICTURE BOOK: VARIOUS PICTURES

40 FULL COLOR IMAGES

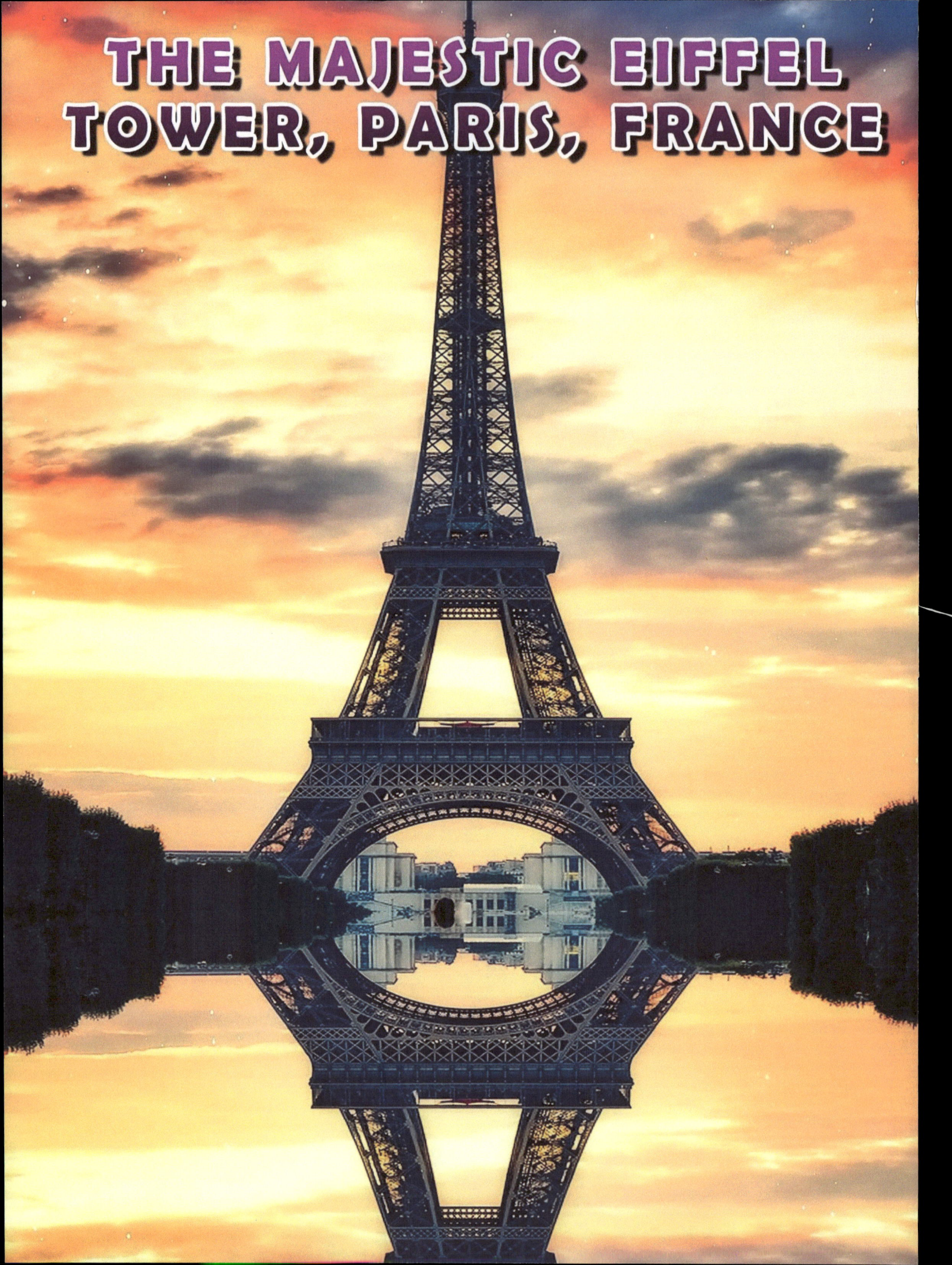

THE MAJESTIC EIFFEL TOWER, PARIS, FRANCE

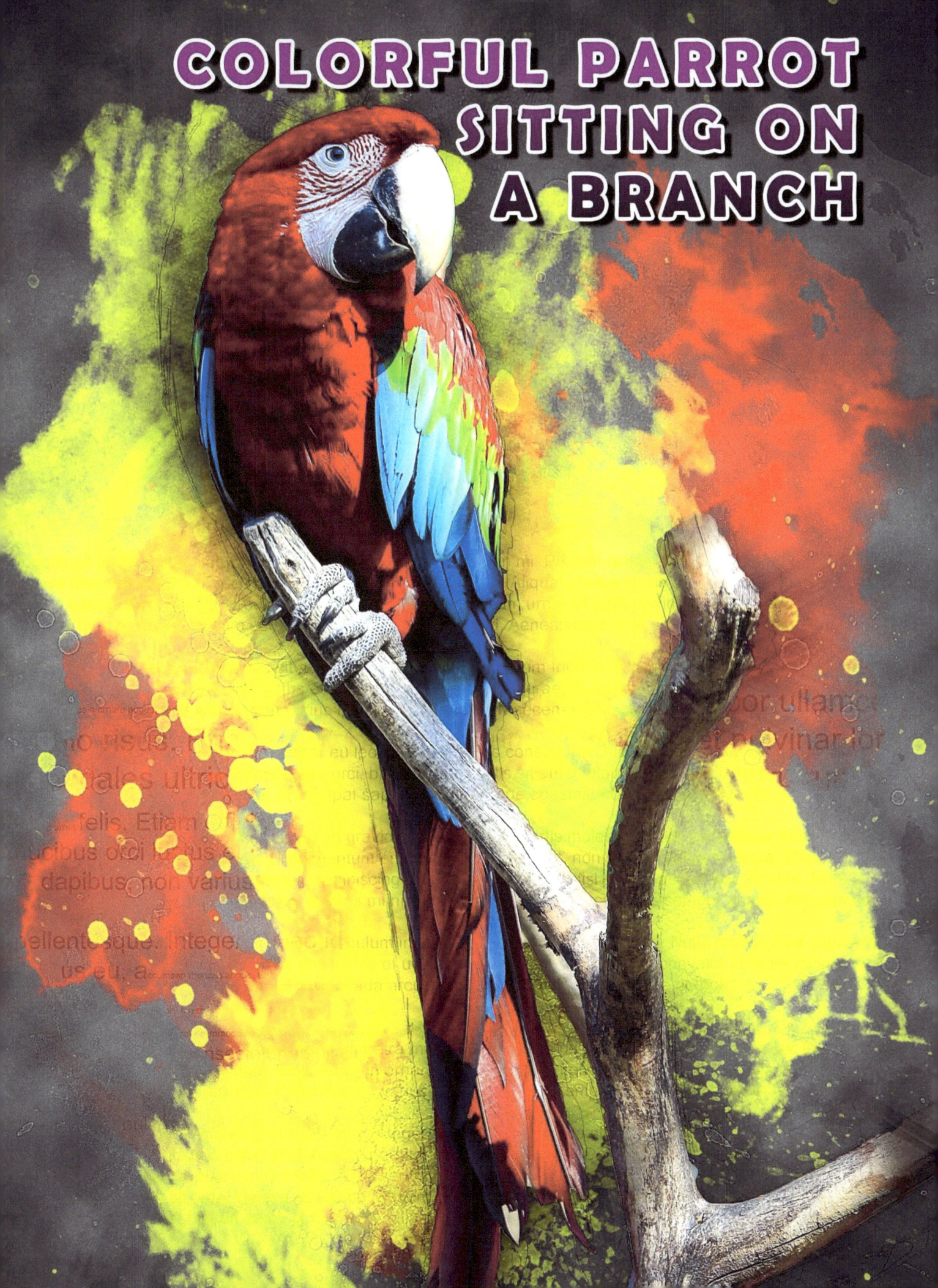

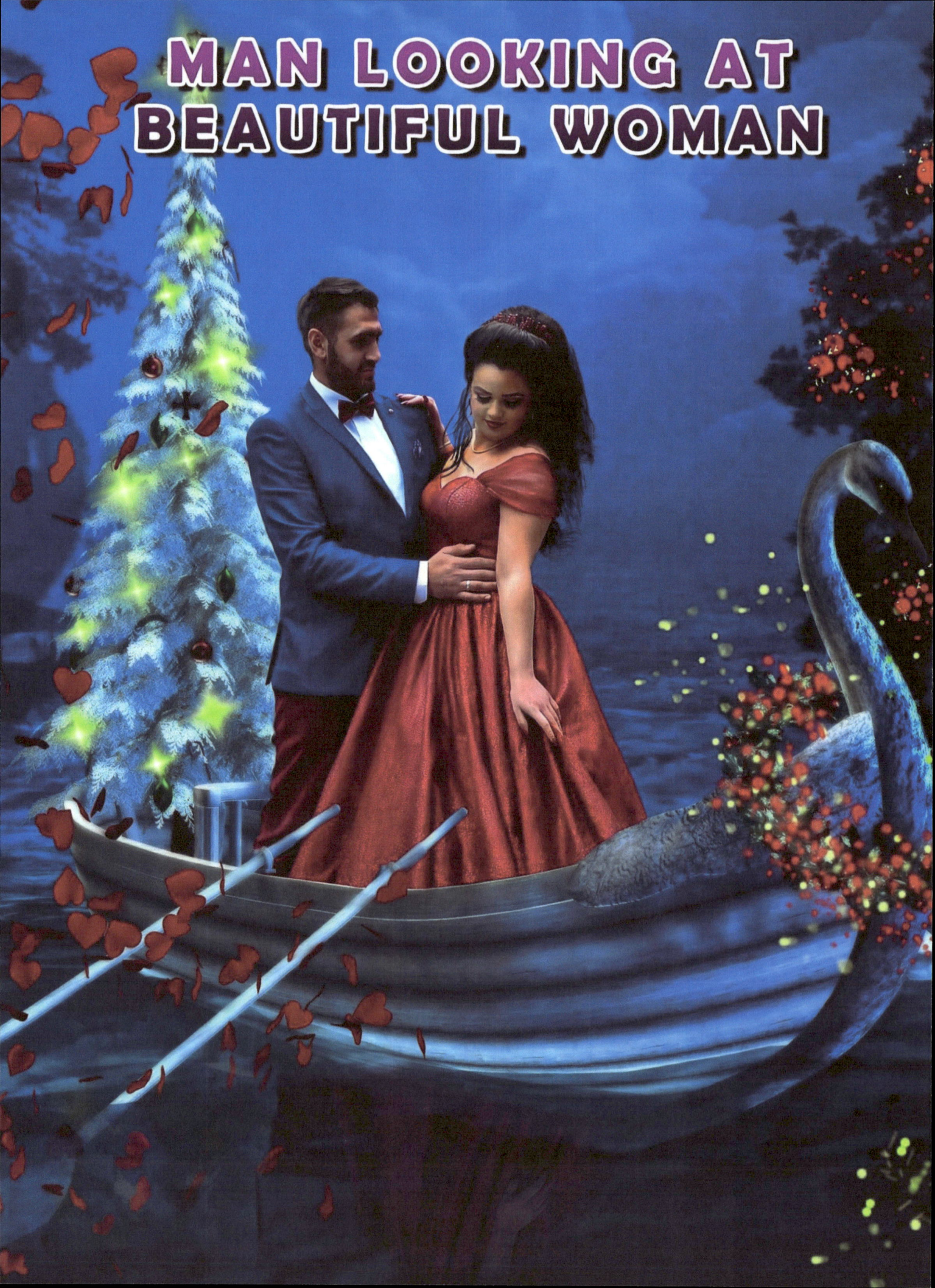

MAN LOOKING AT BEAUTIFUL WOMAN

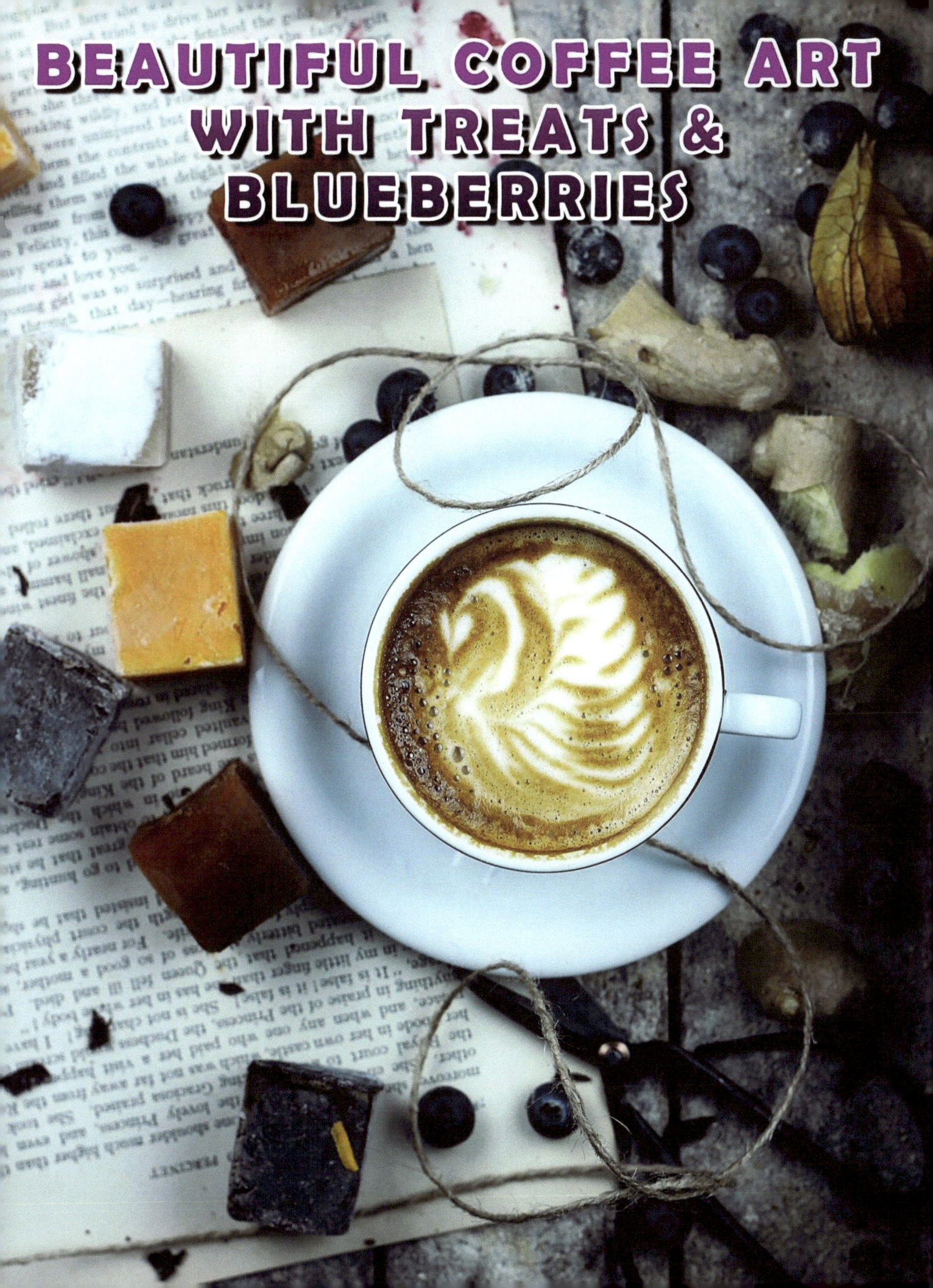

BEAUTIFUL COFFEE ART WITH TREATS & BLUEBERRIES

LITTLE GIRL IN
BEAUTIFUL WHITE DRESS

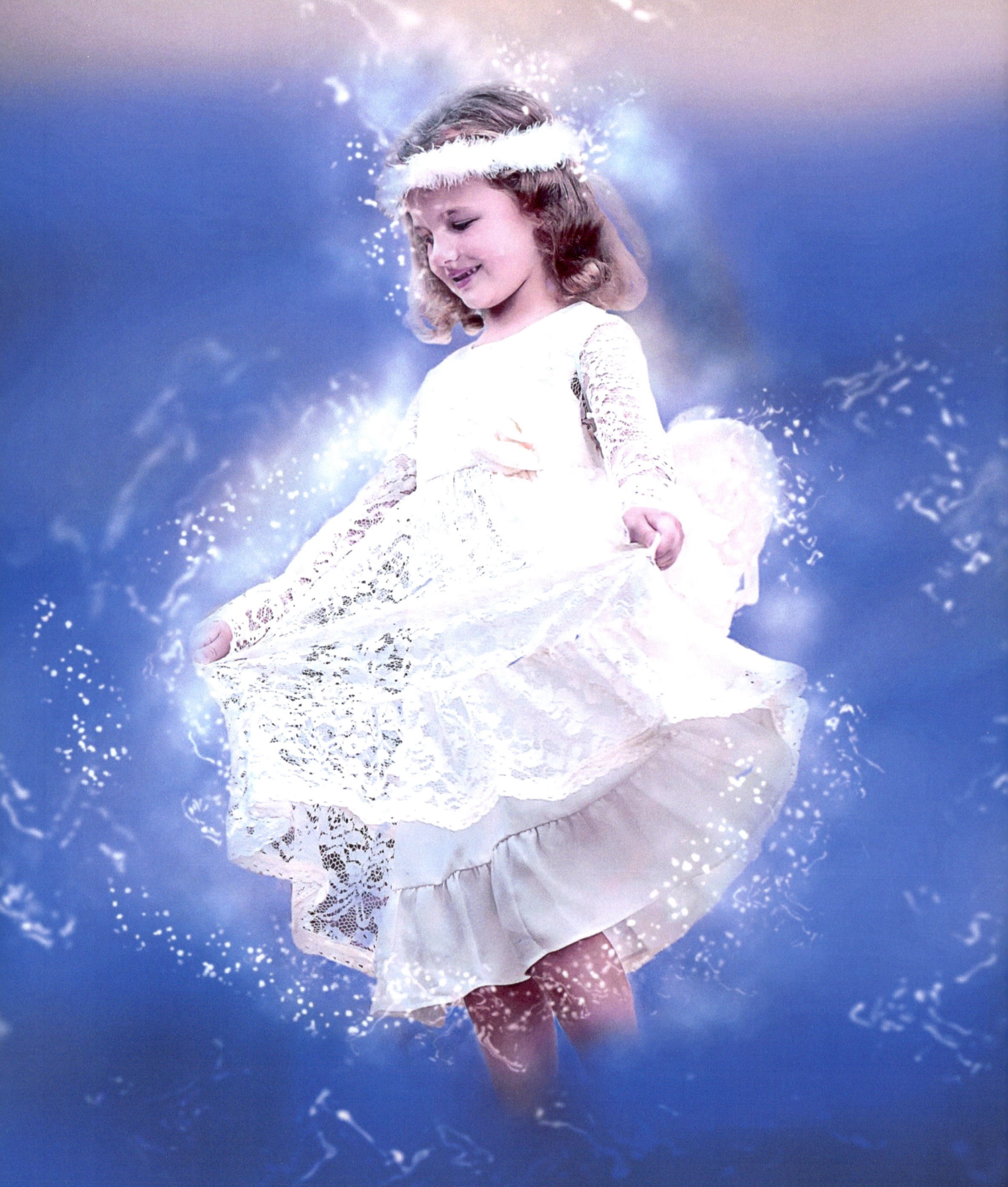

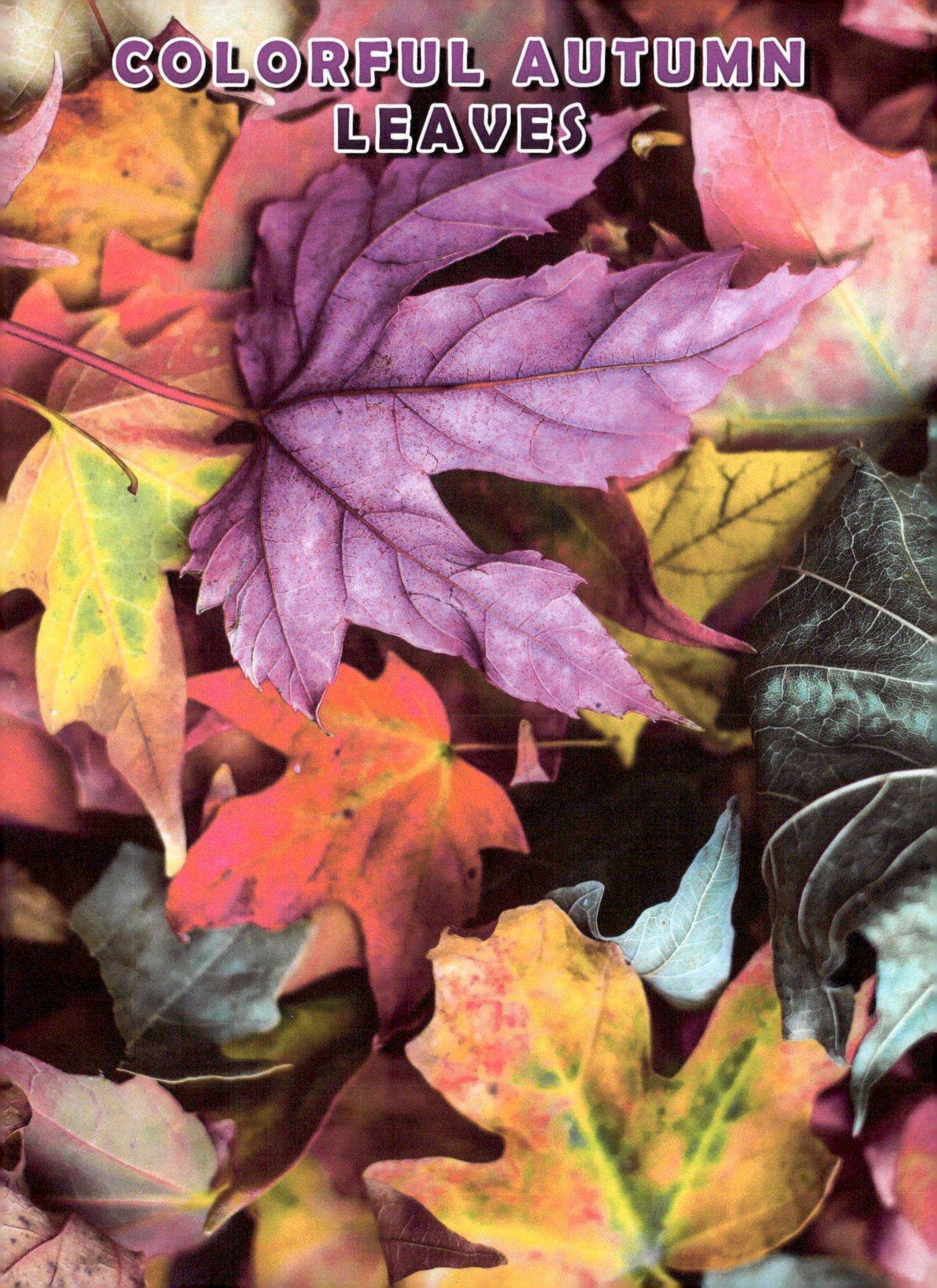

COLORFUL AUTUMN LEAVES

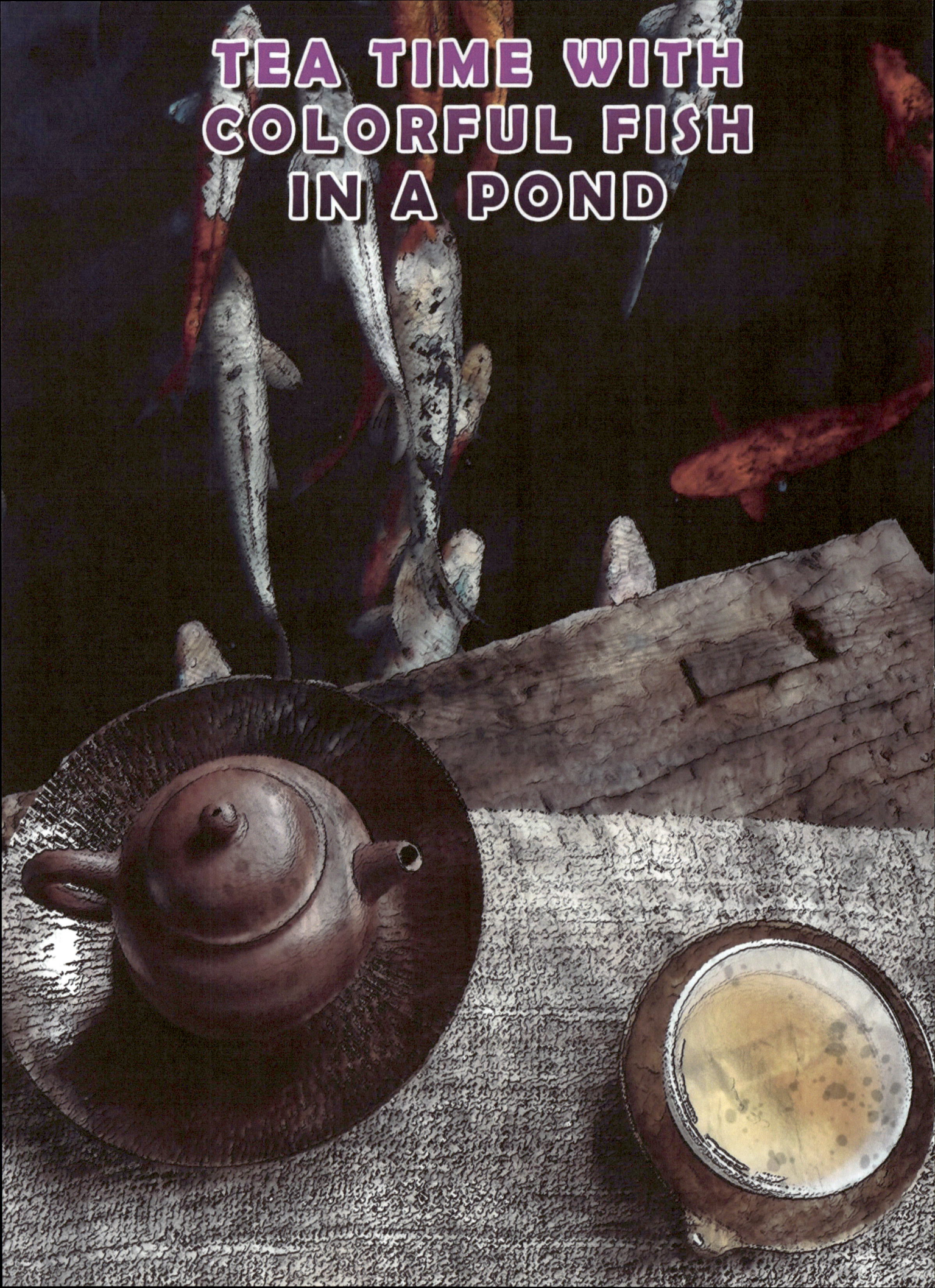

TEA TIME WITH COLORFUL FISH IN A POND

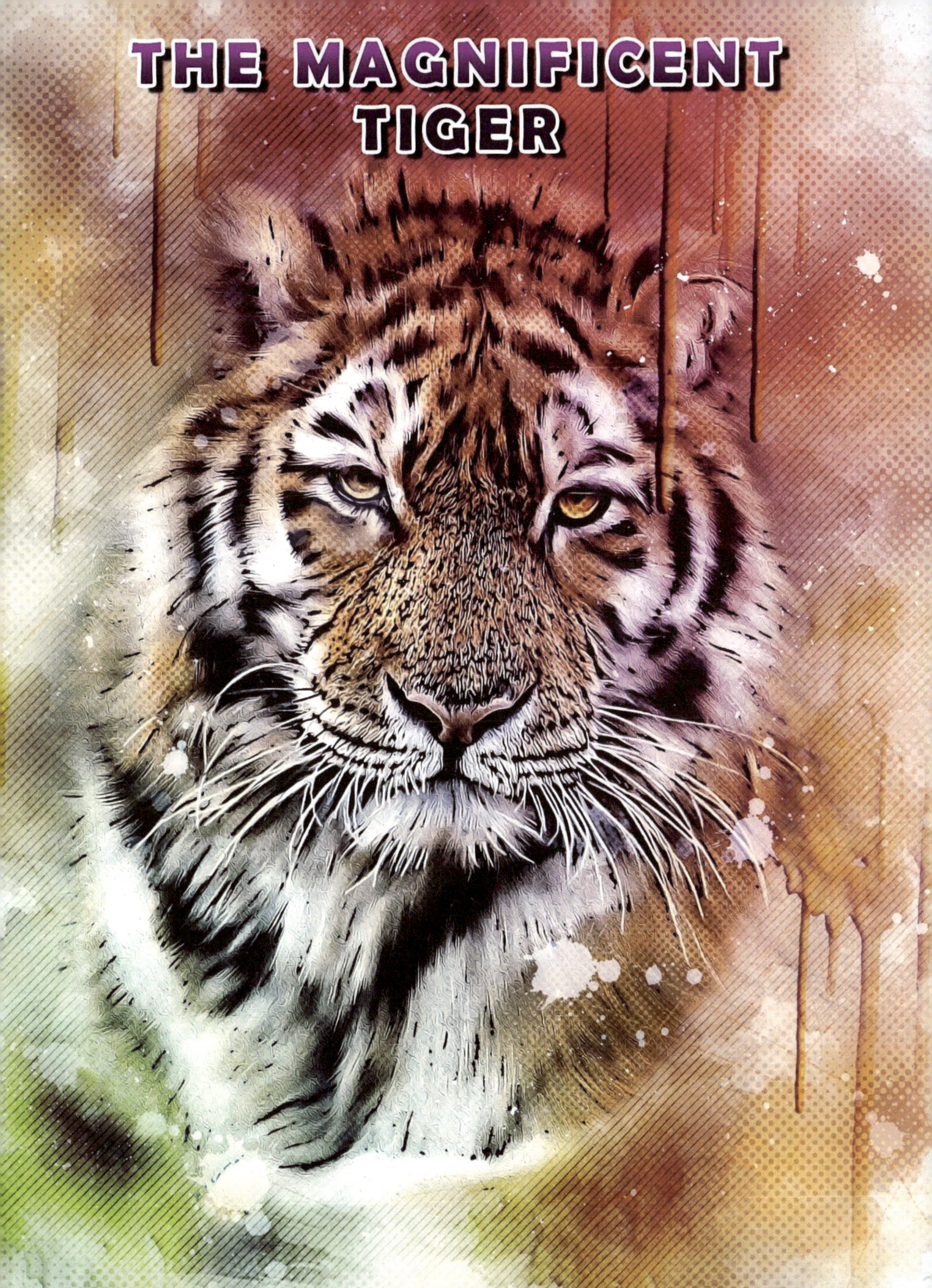

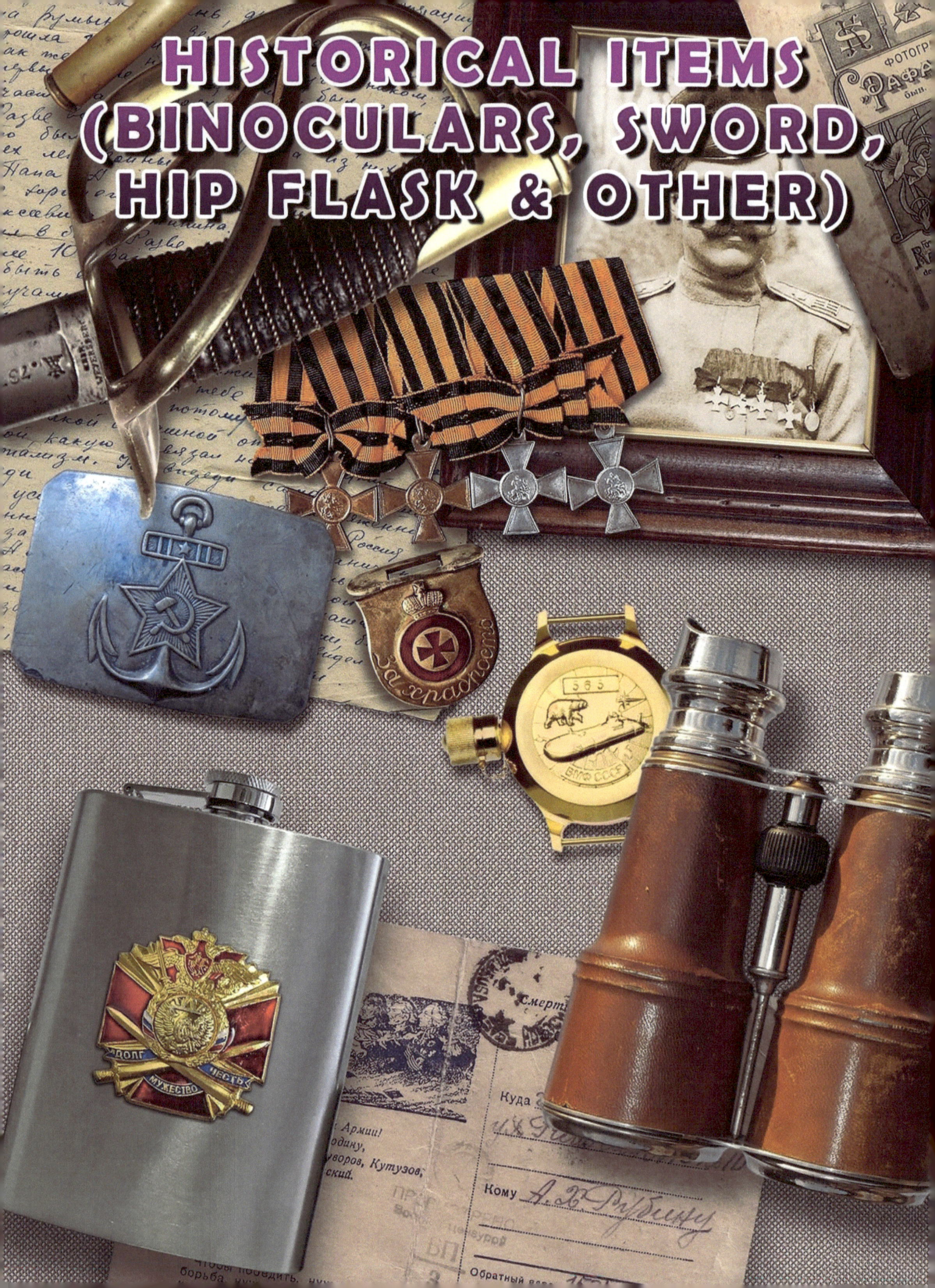

HISTORICAL ITEMS (BINOCULARS, SWORD, HIP FLASK & OTHER)

THE DETECTIVE DOG

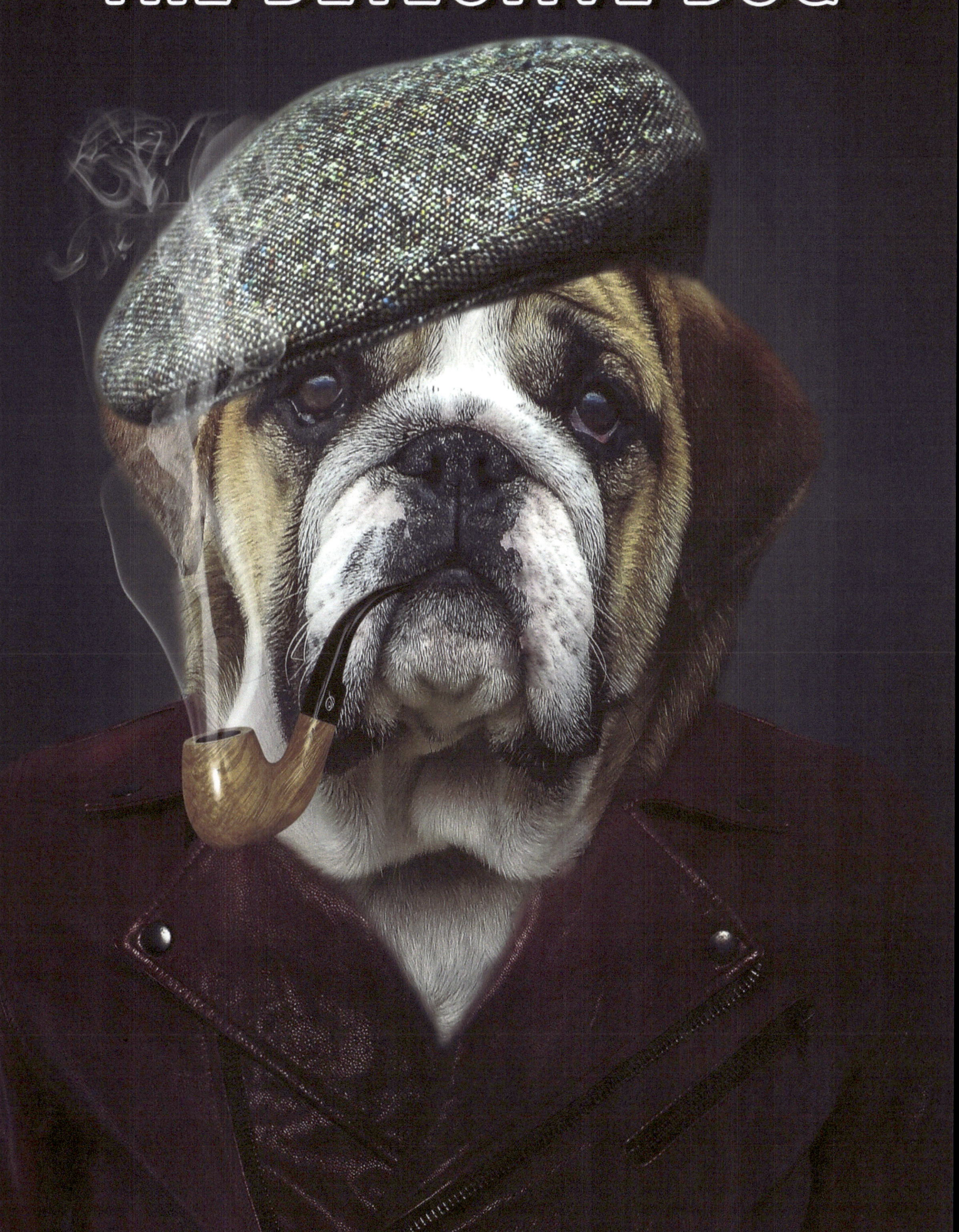

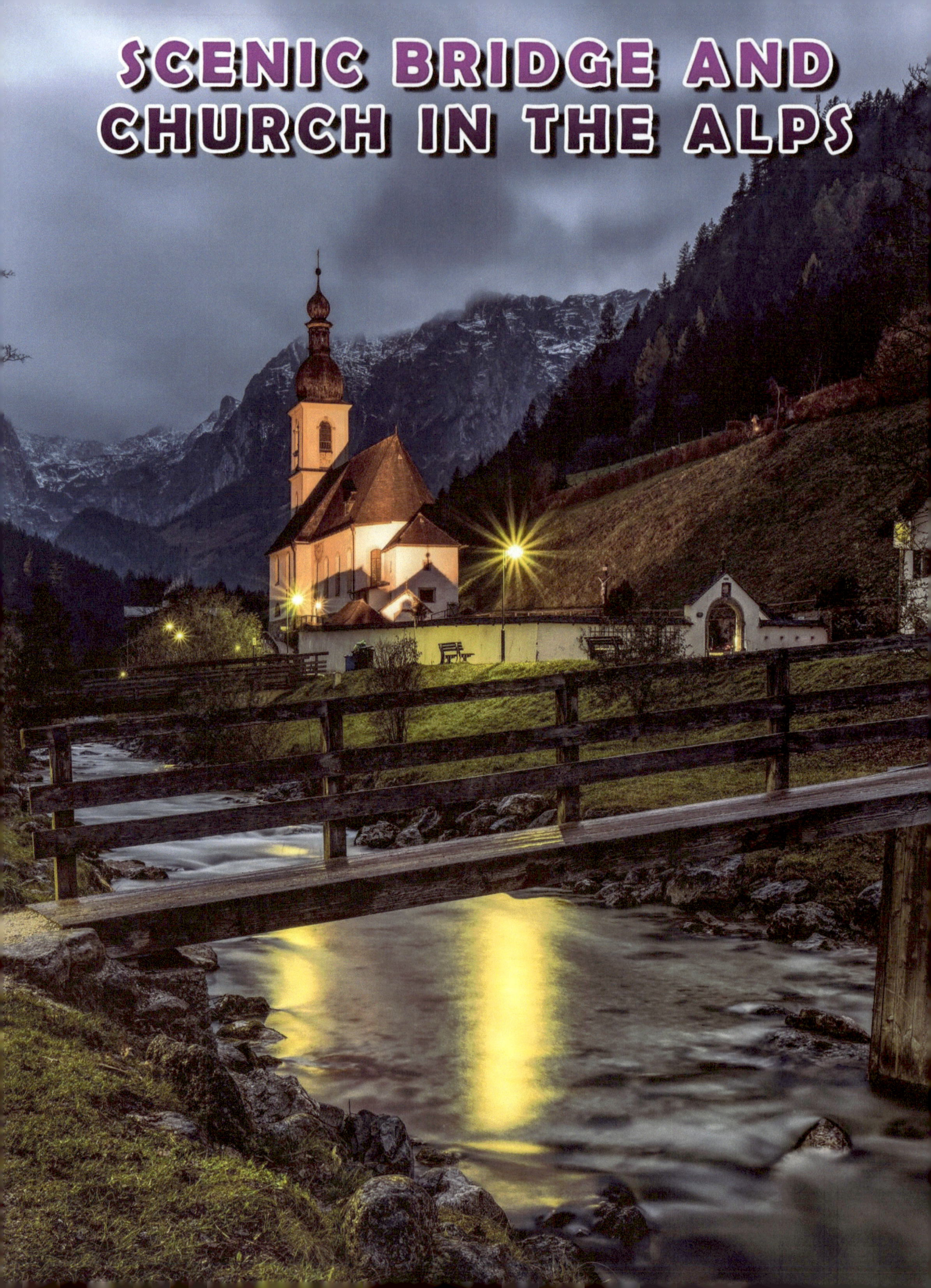

SCENIC BRIDGE AND CHURCH IN THE ALPS

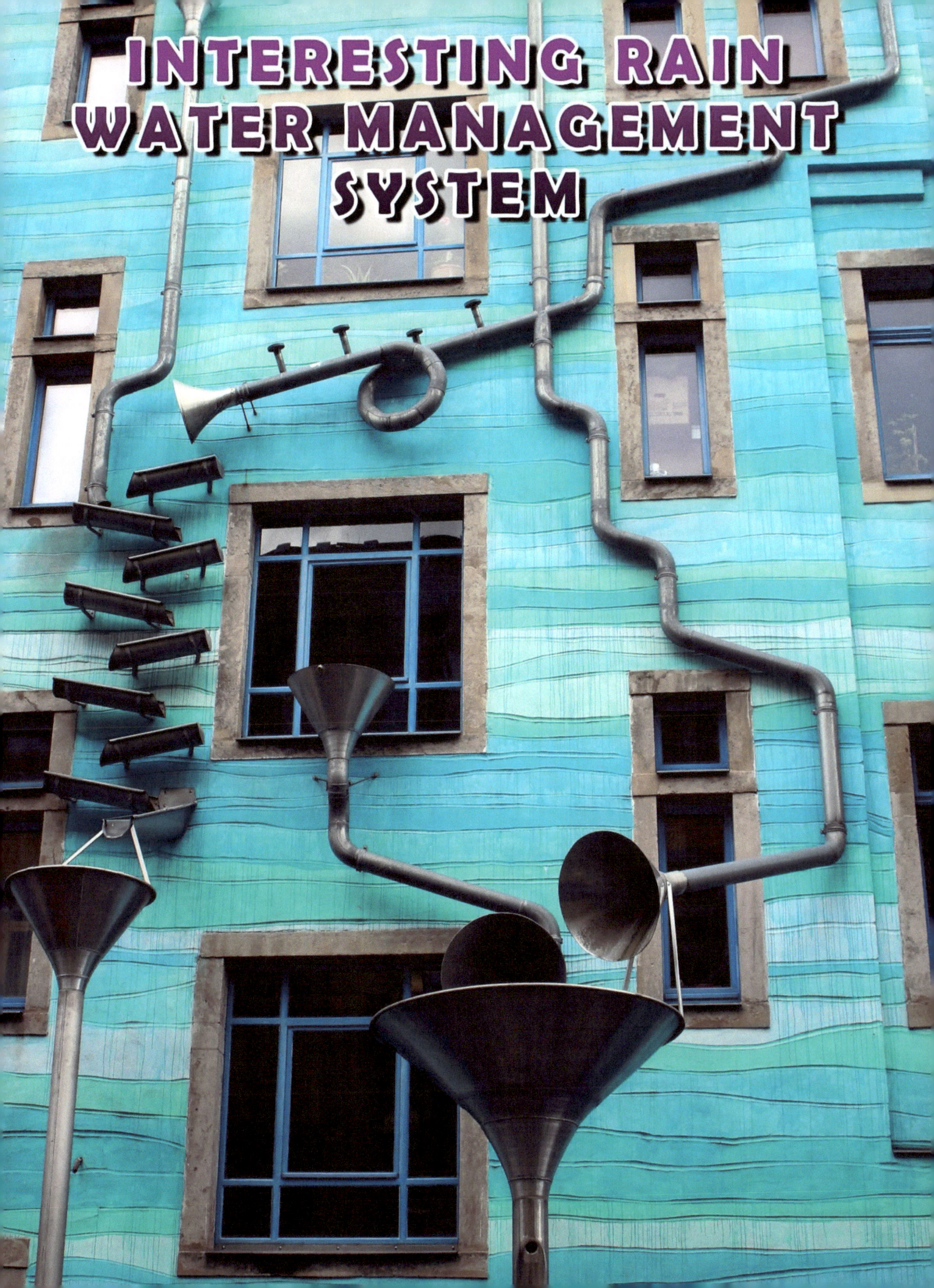

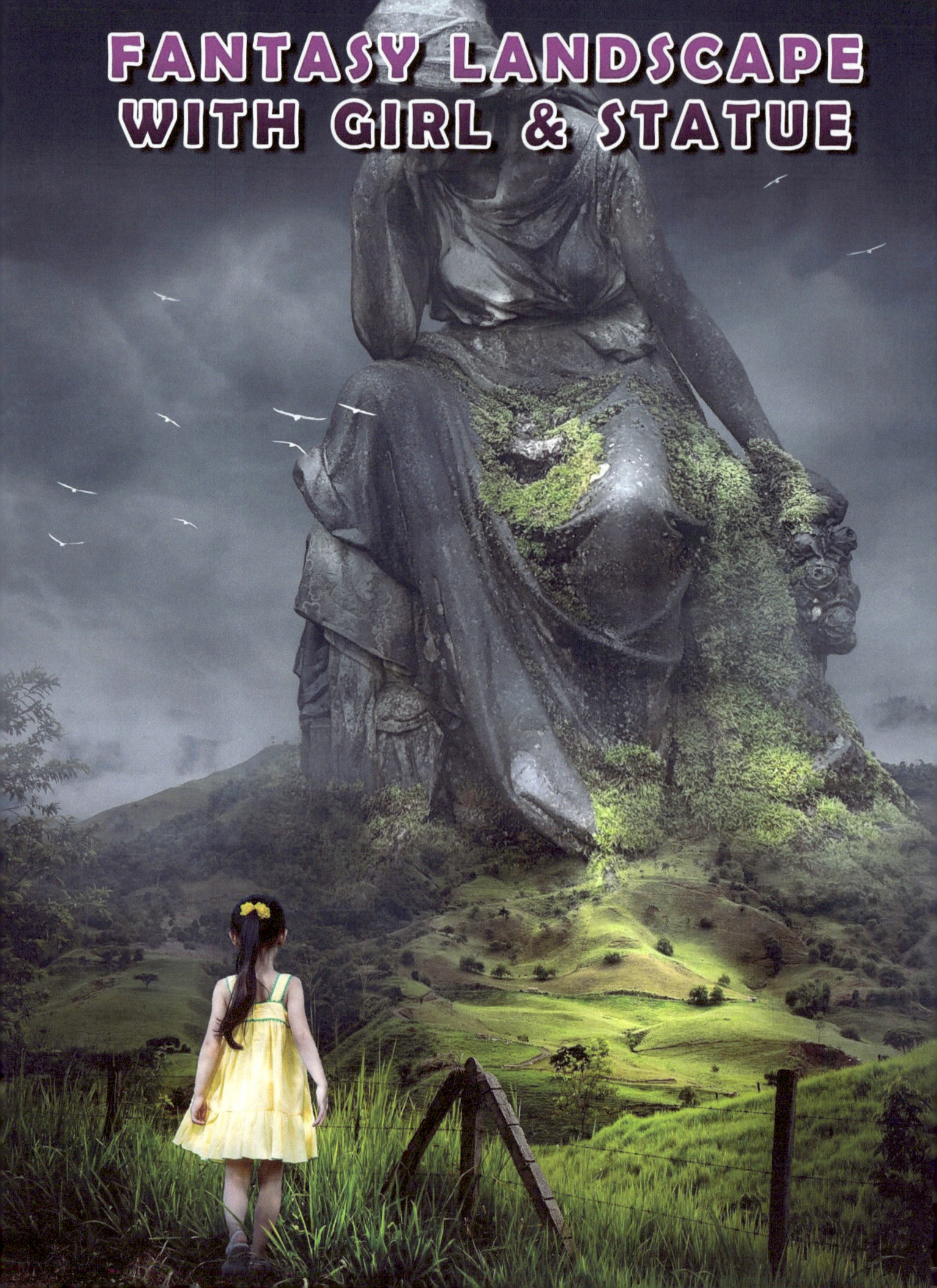

FANTASY LANDSCAPE
WITH GIRL & STATUE

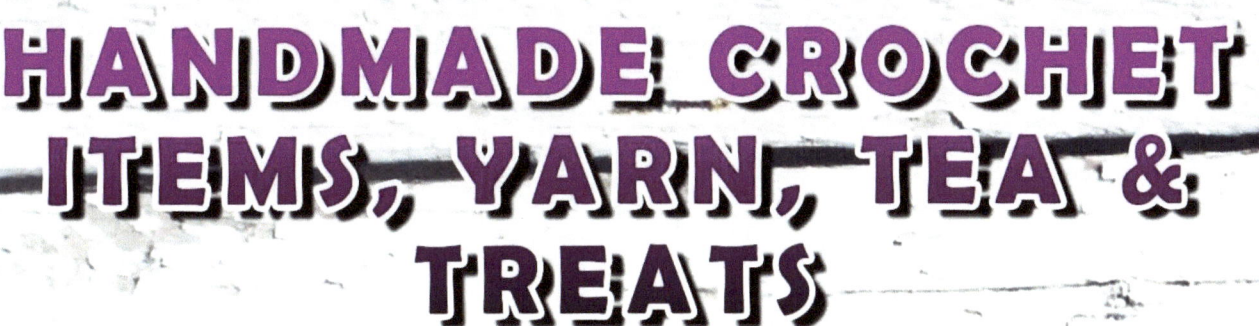

HANDMADE CROCHET ITEMS, YARN, TEA & TREATS

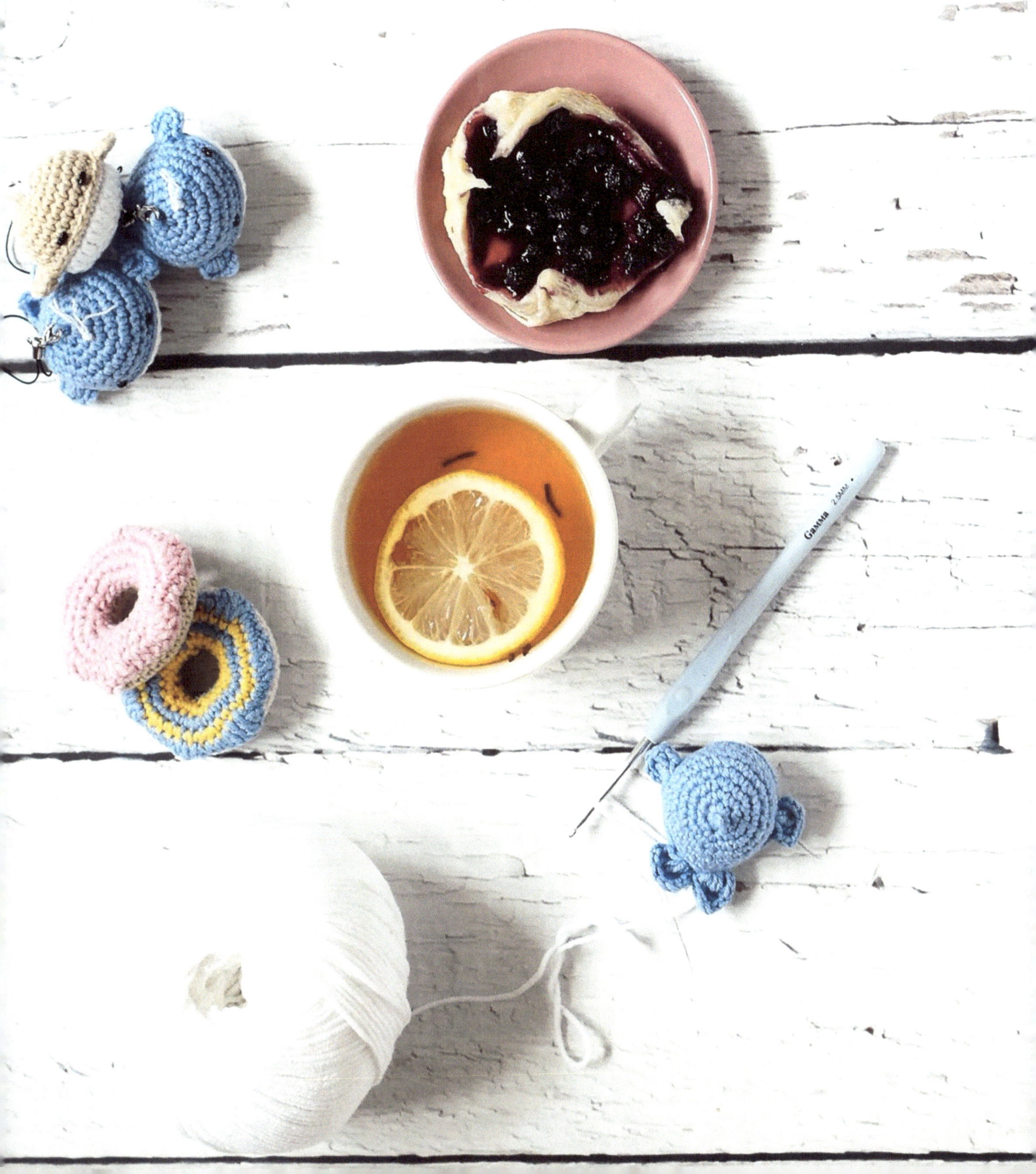

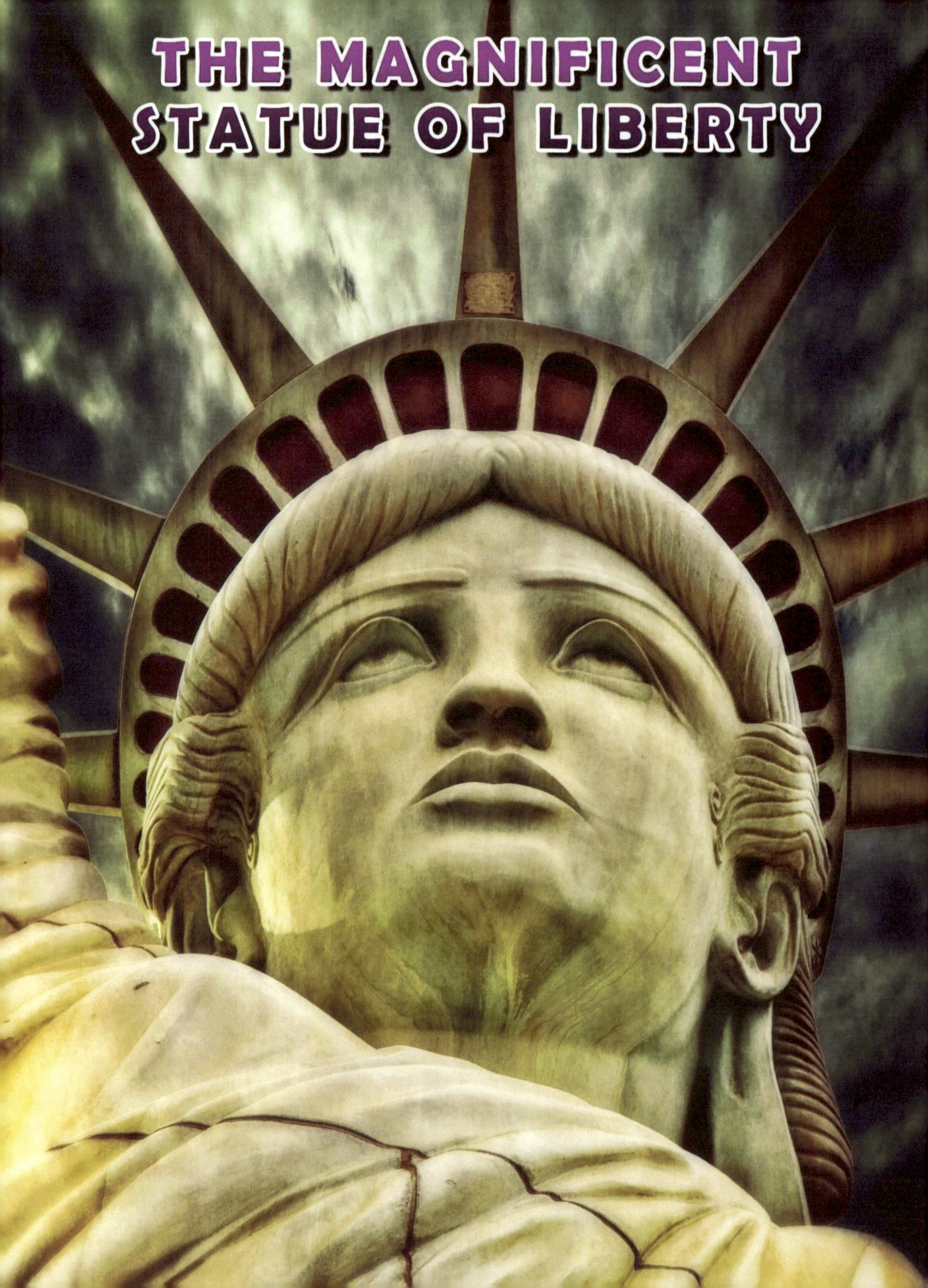

THE MAGNIFICENT STATUE OF LIBERTY

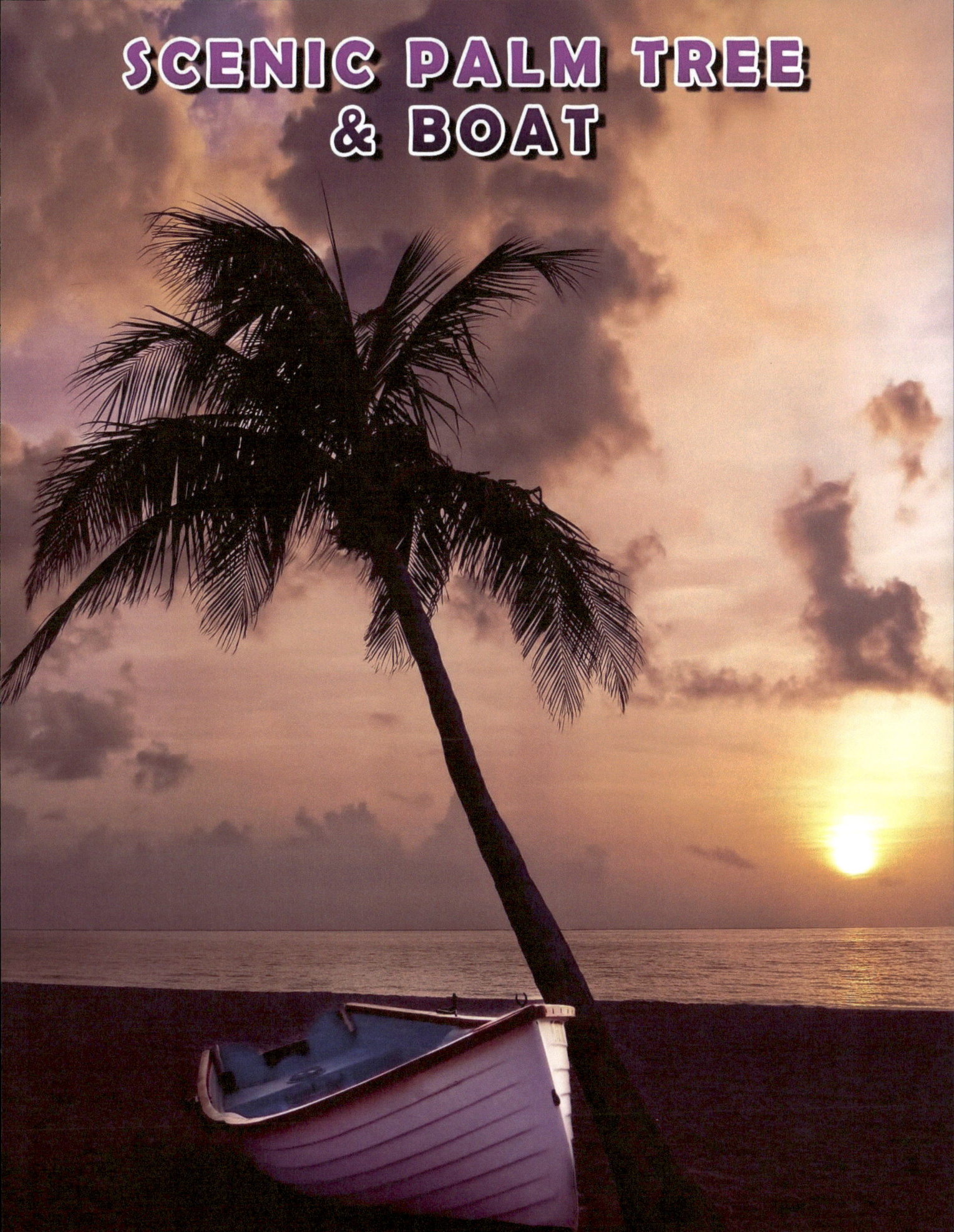

SCENIC PALM TREE & BOAT

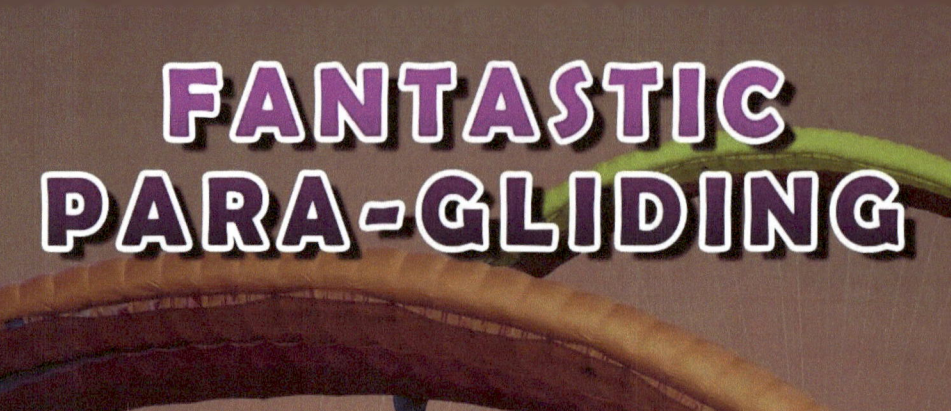

FANTASTIC PARA-GLIDING

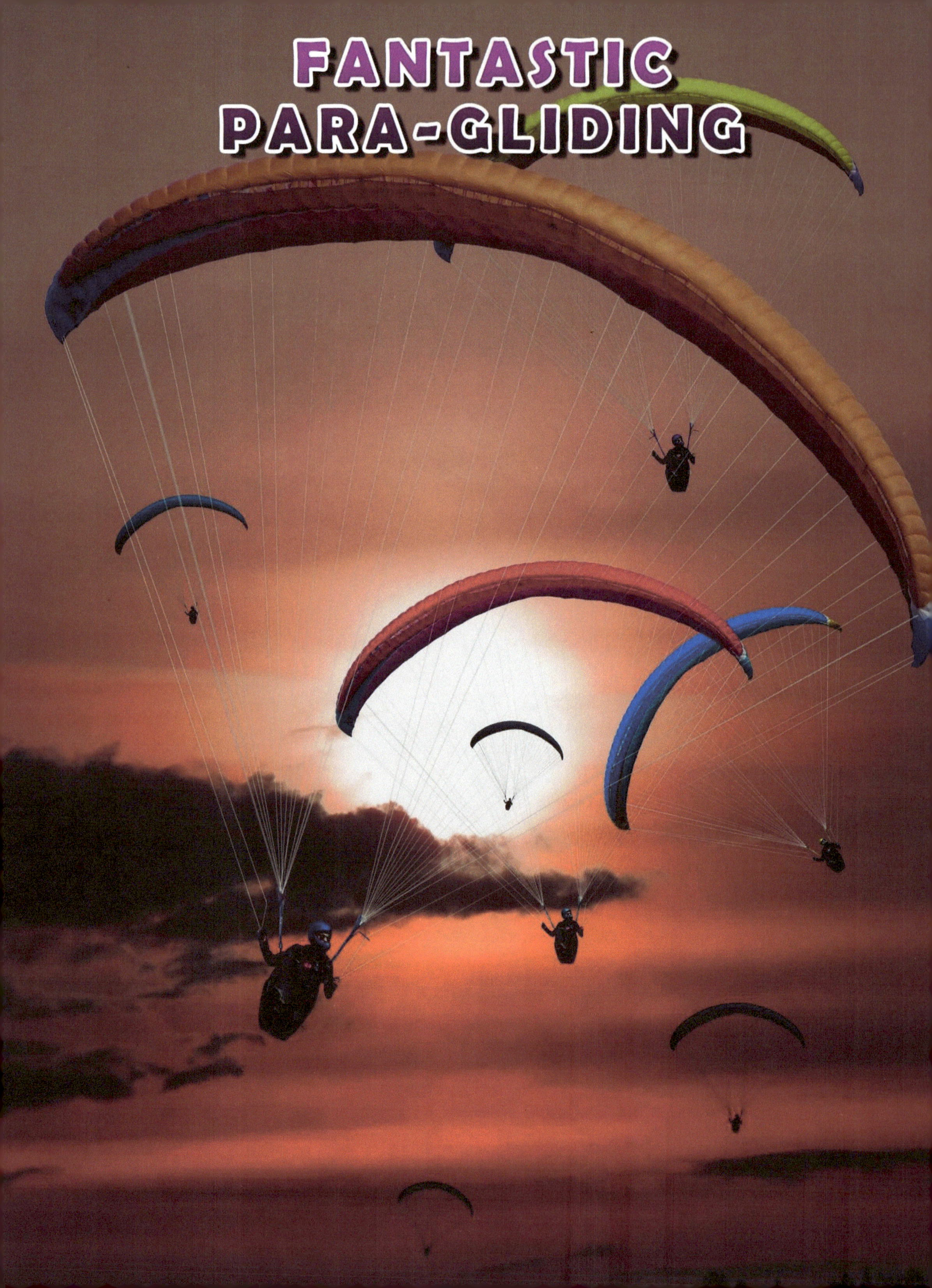

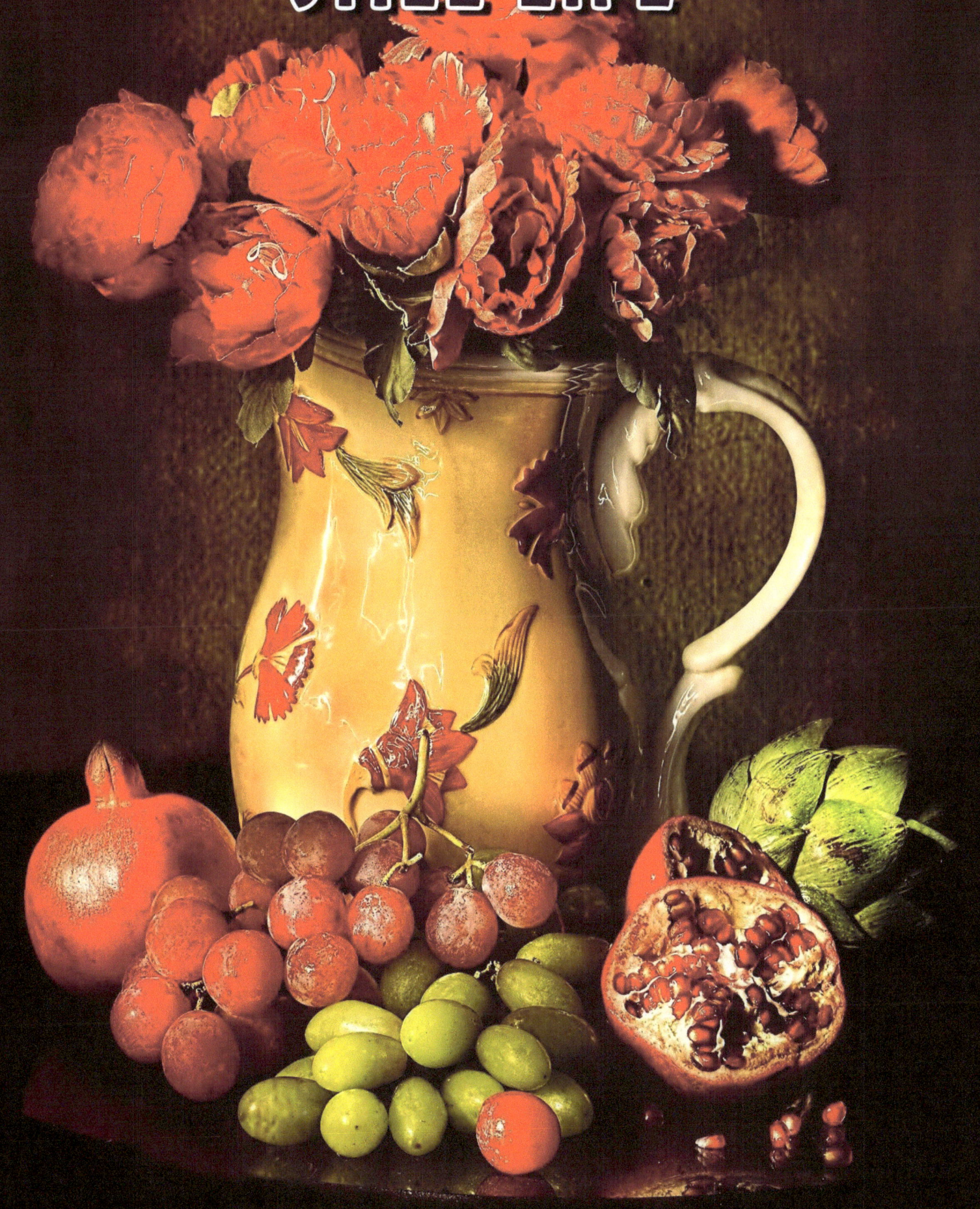

A BEAUTIFUL FLOWER
STILL LIFE

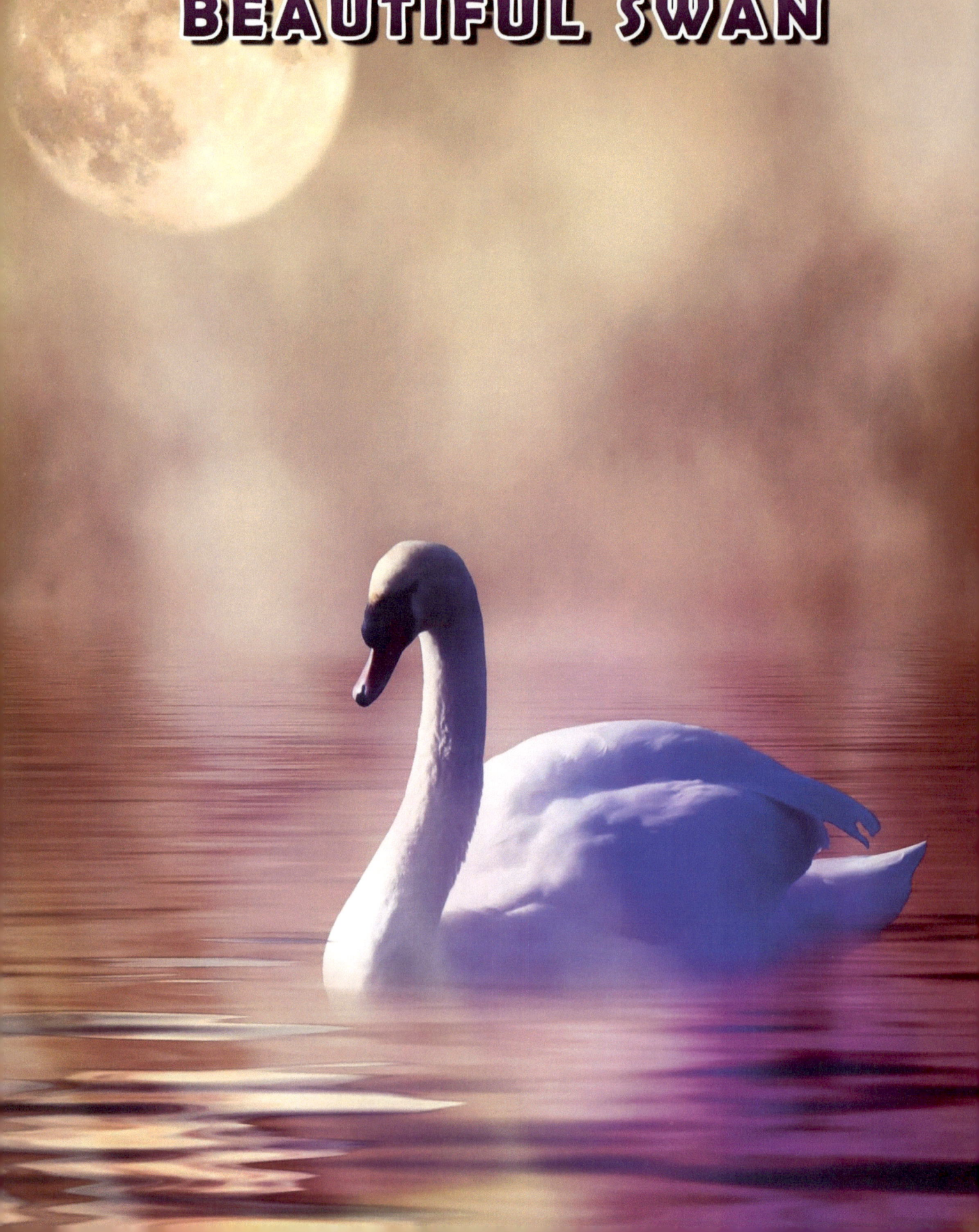

A FULL MOON AND A BEAUTIFUL SWAN

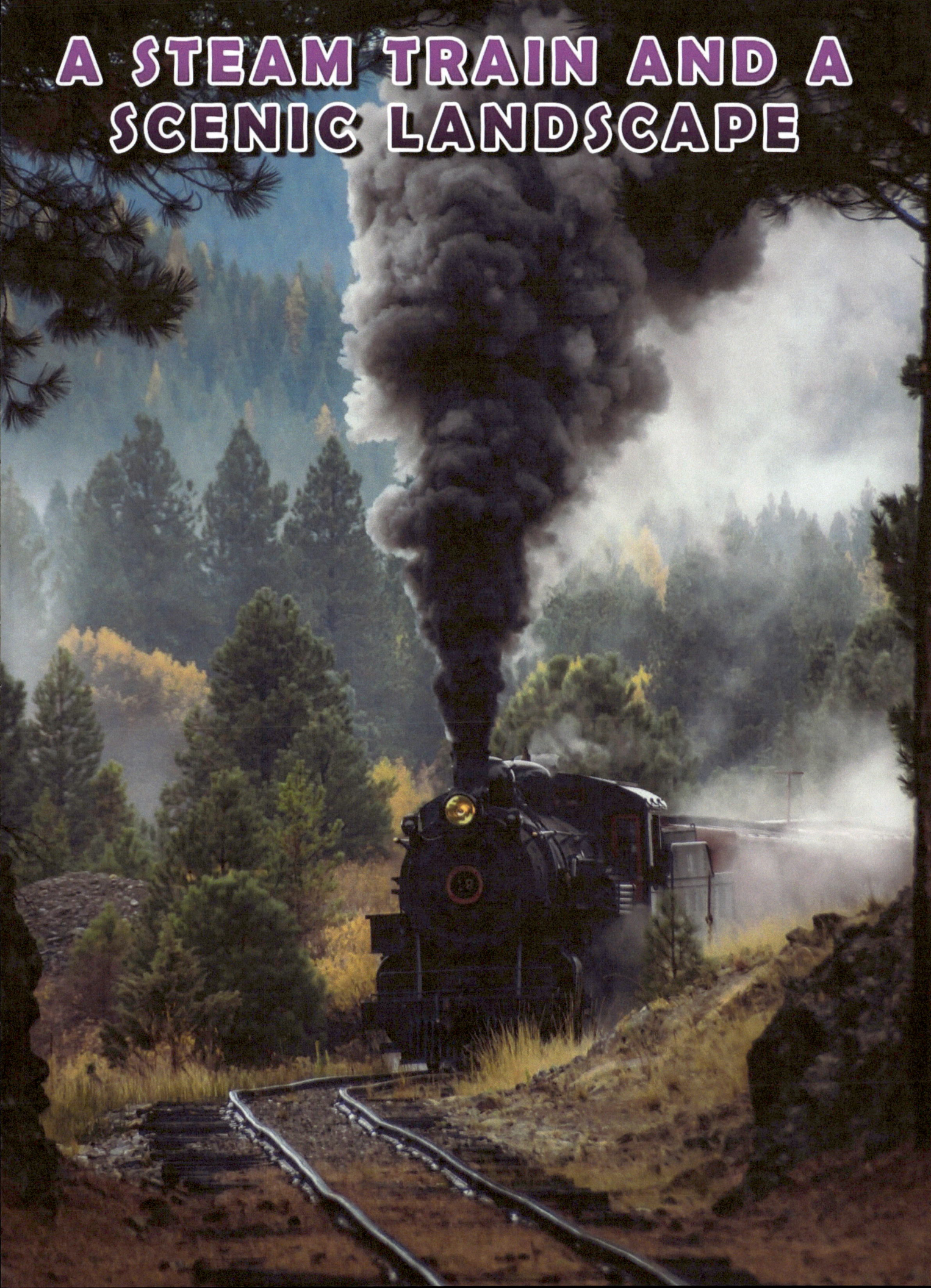

A STEAM TRAIN AND A SCENIC LANDSCAPE

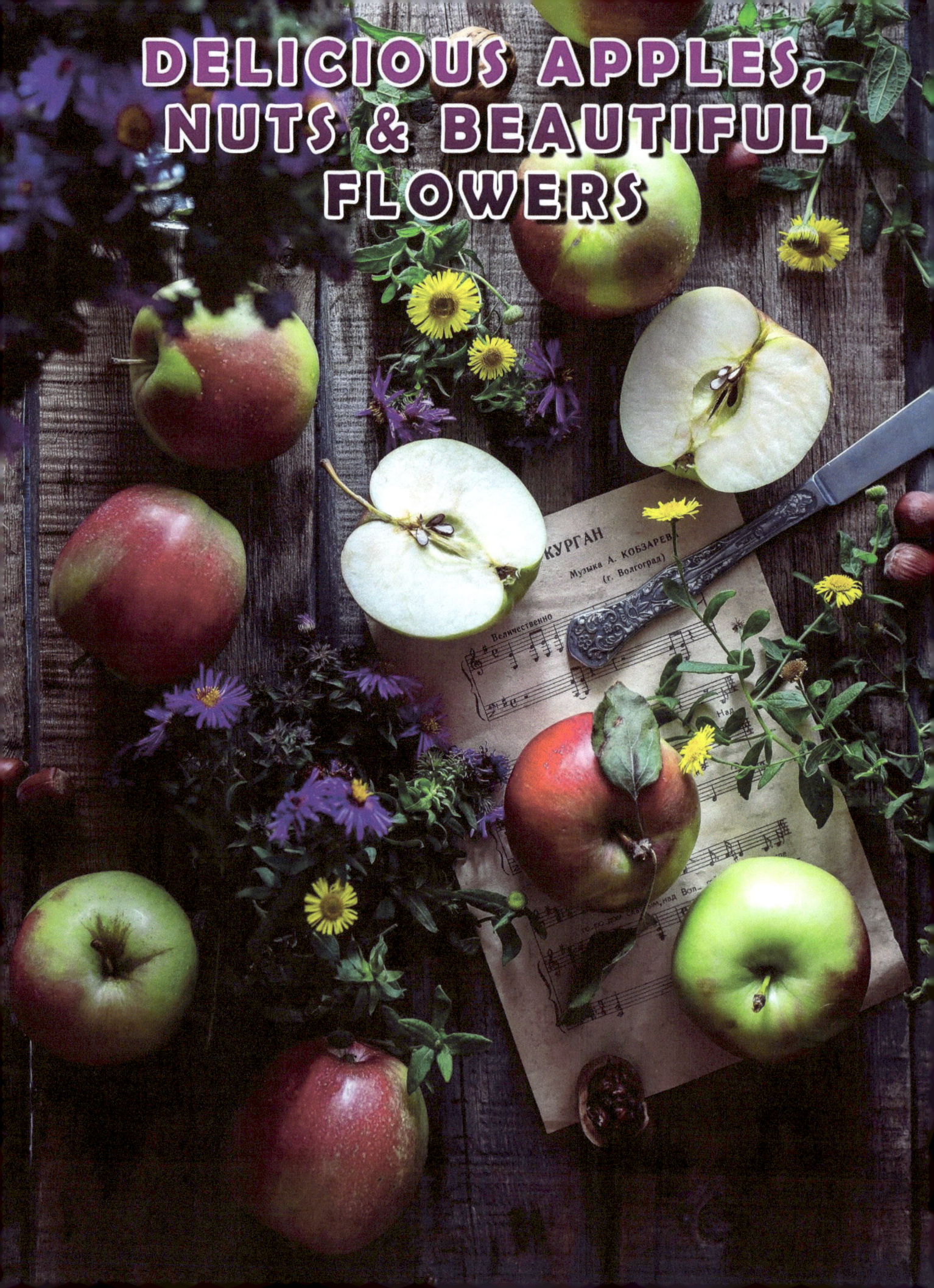

DELICIOUS APPLES, NUTS & BEAUTIFUL FLOWERS

CLASSIC YELLOW CAR & GUITAR

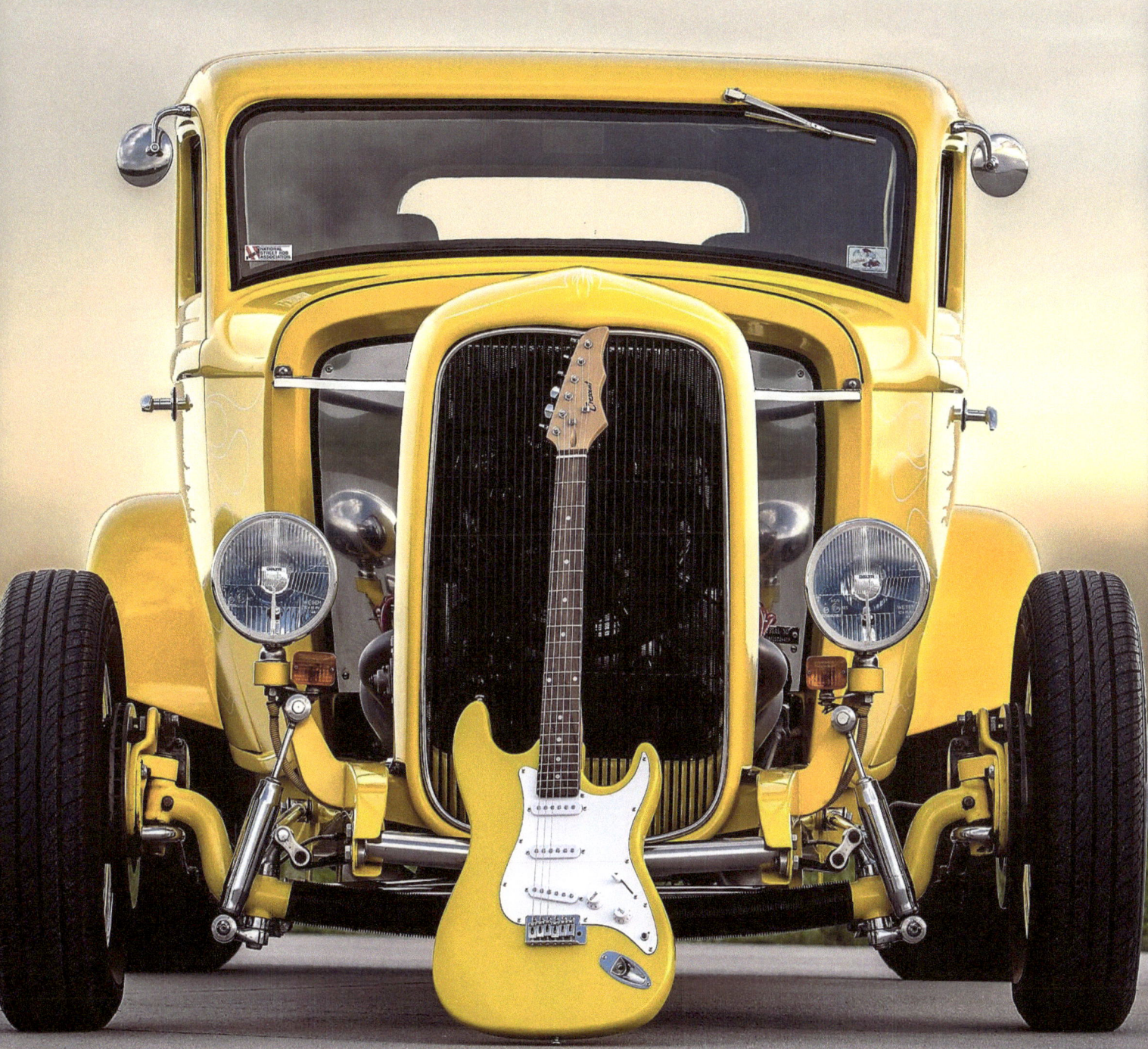

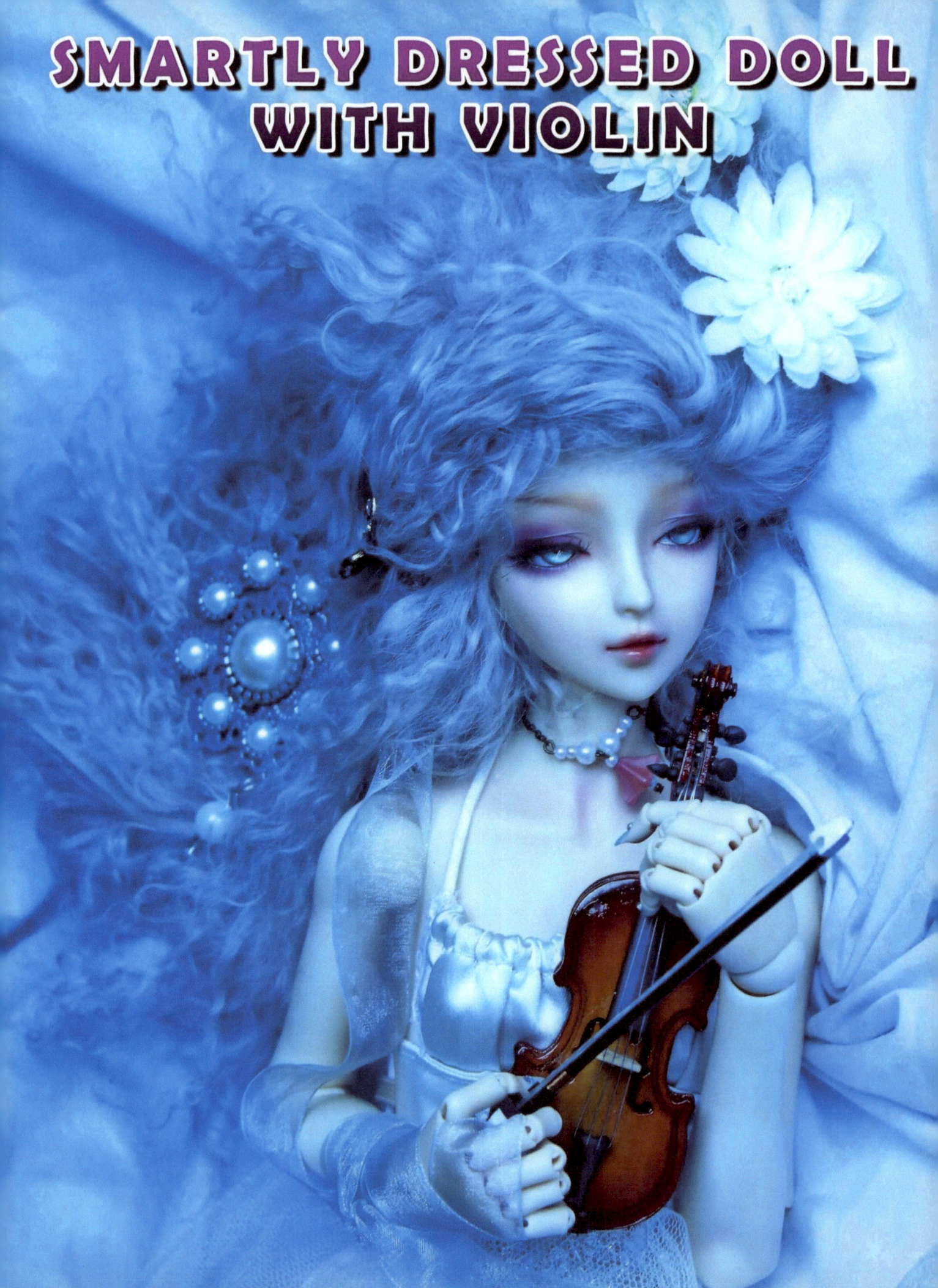

SMARTLY DRESSED DOLL WITH VIOLIN

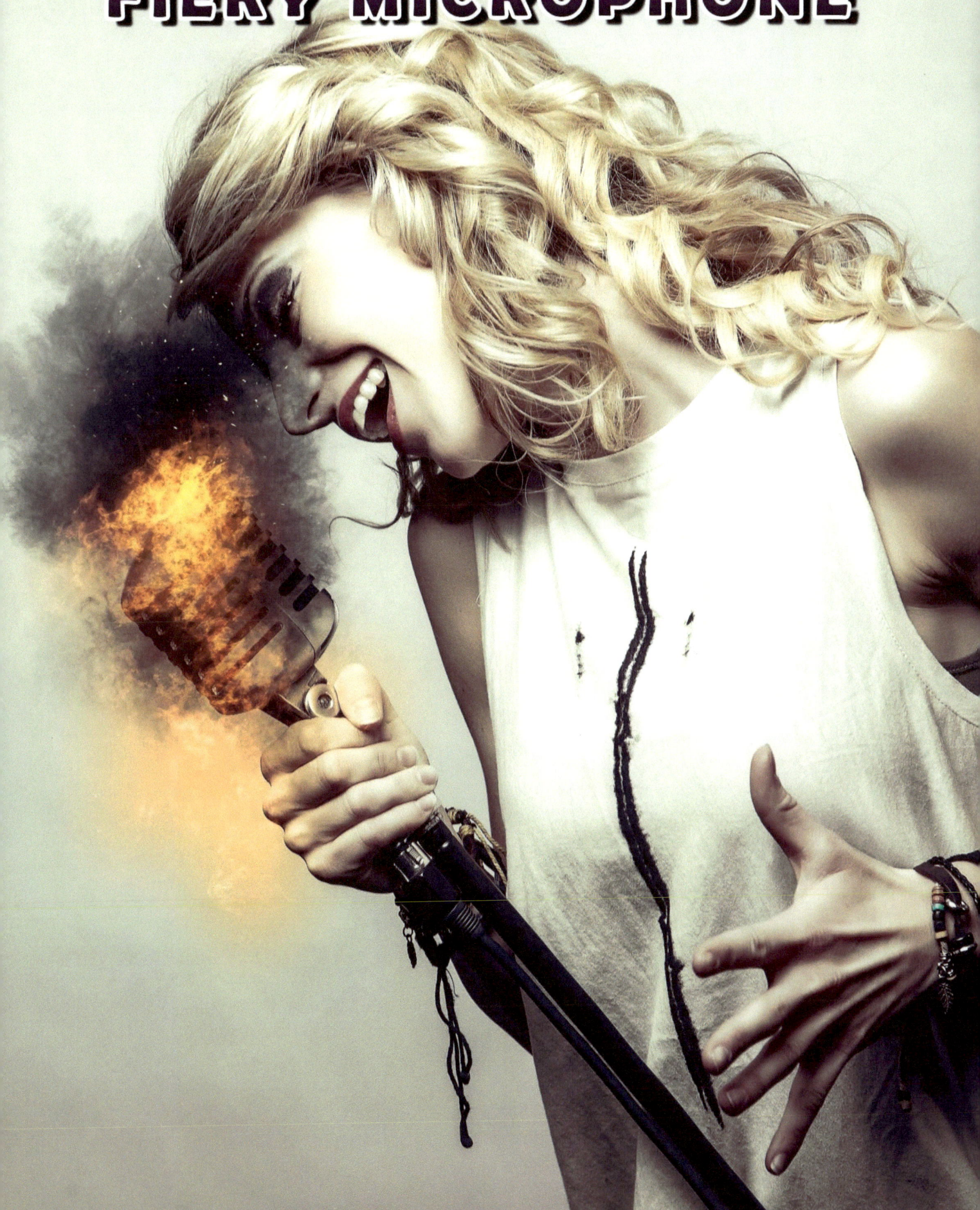

LOVELY LADY WITH FIERY MICROPHONE

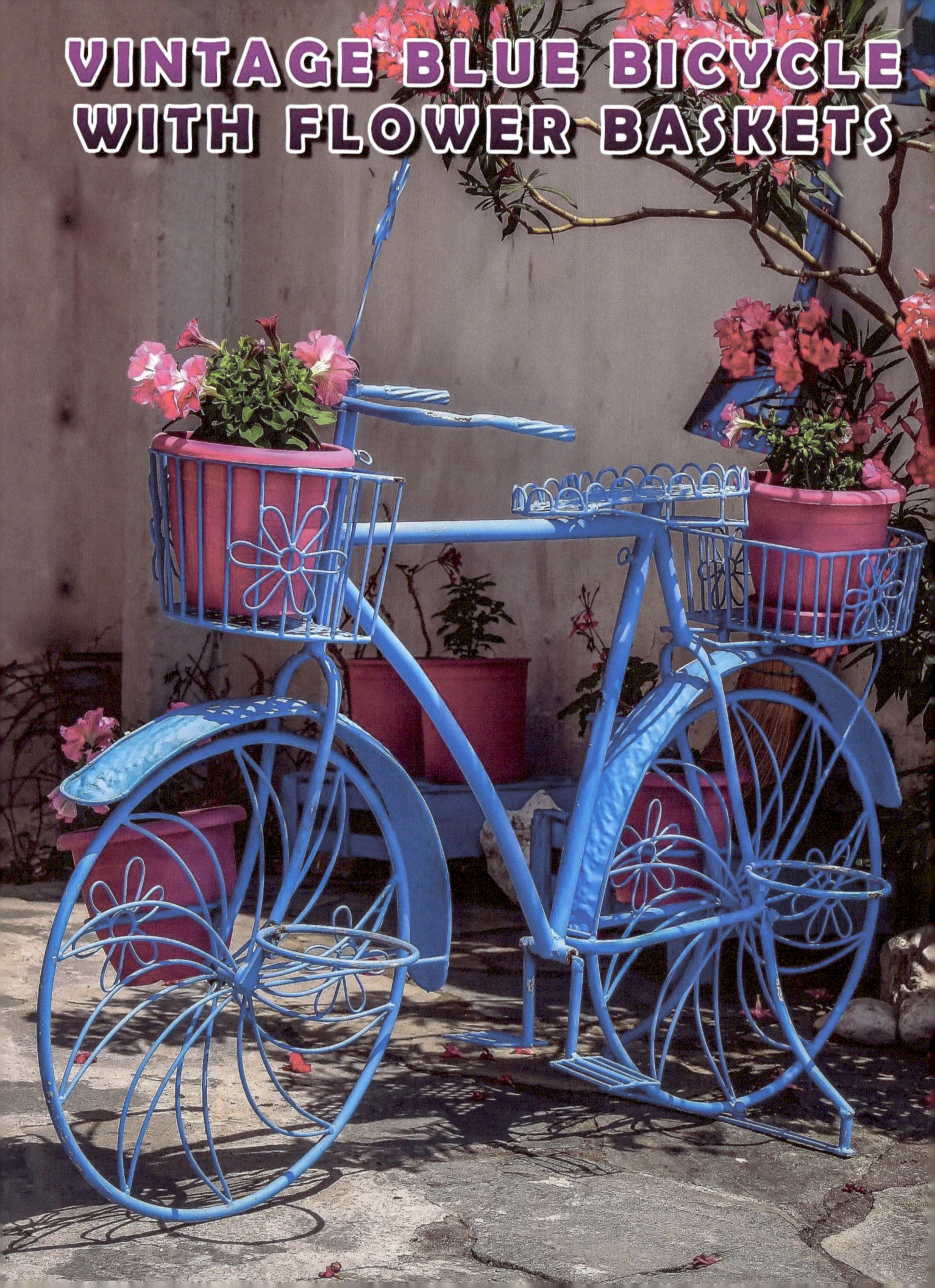

VINTAGE BLUE BICYCLE WITH FLOWER BASKETS

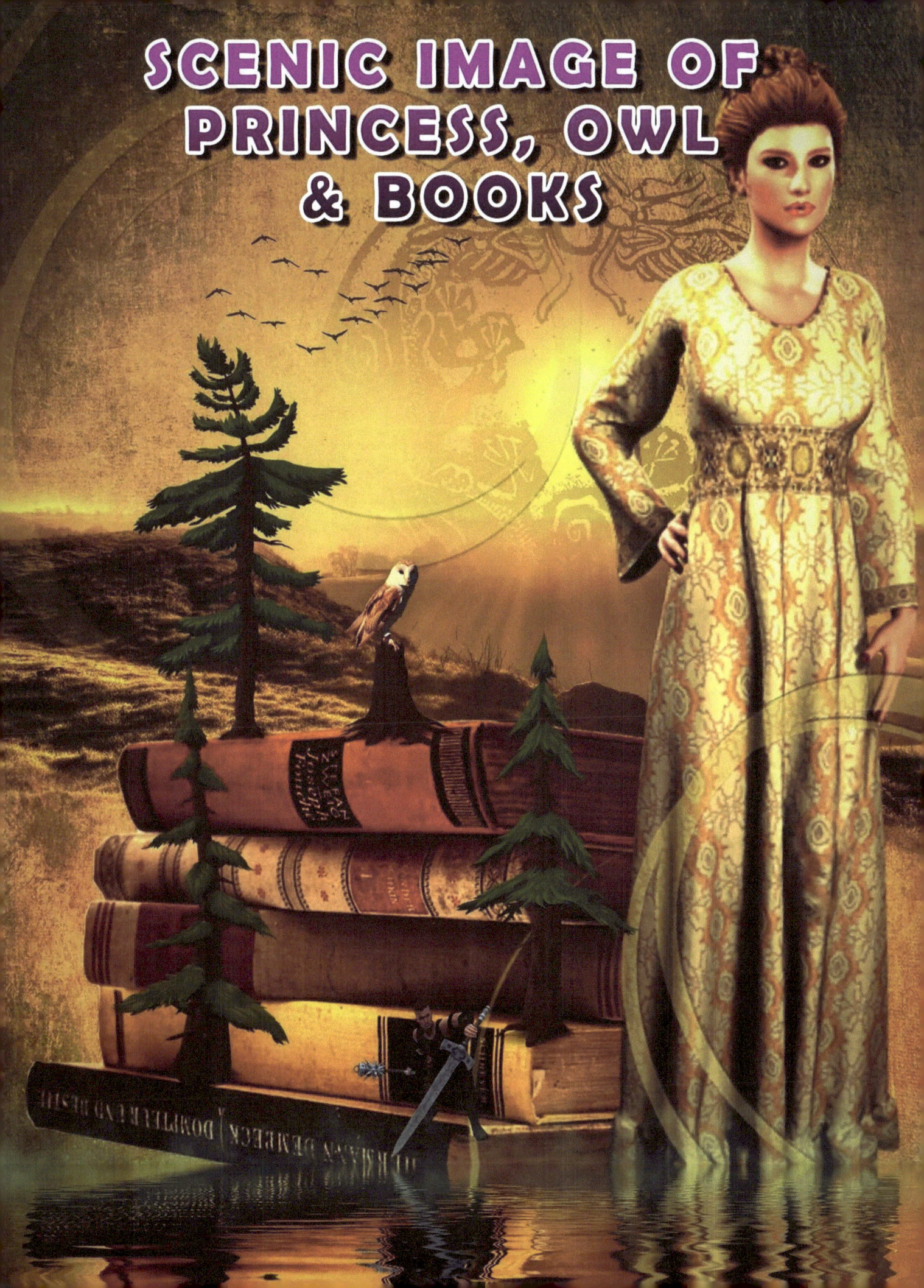

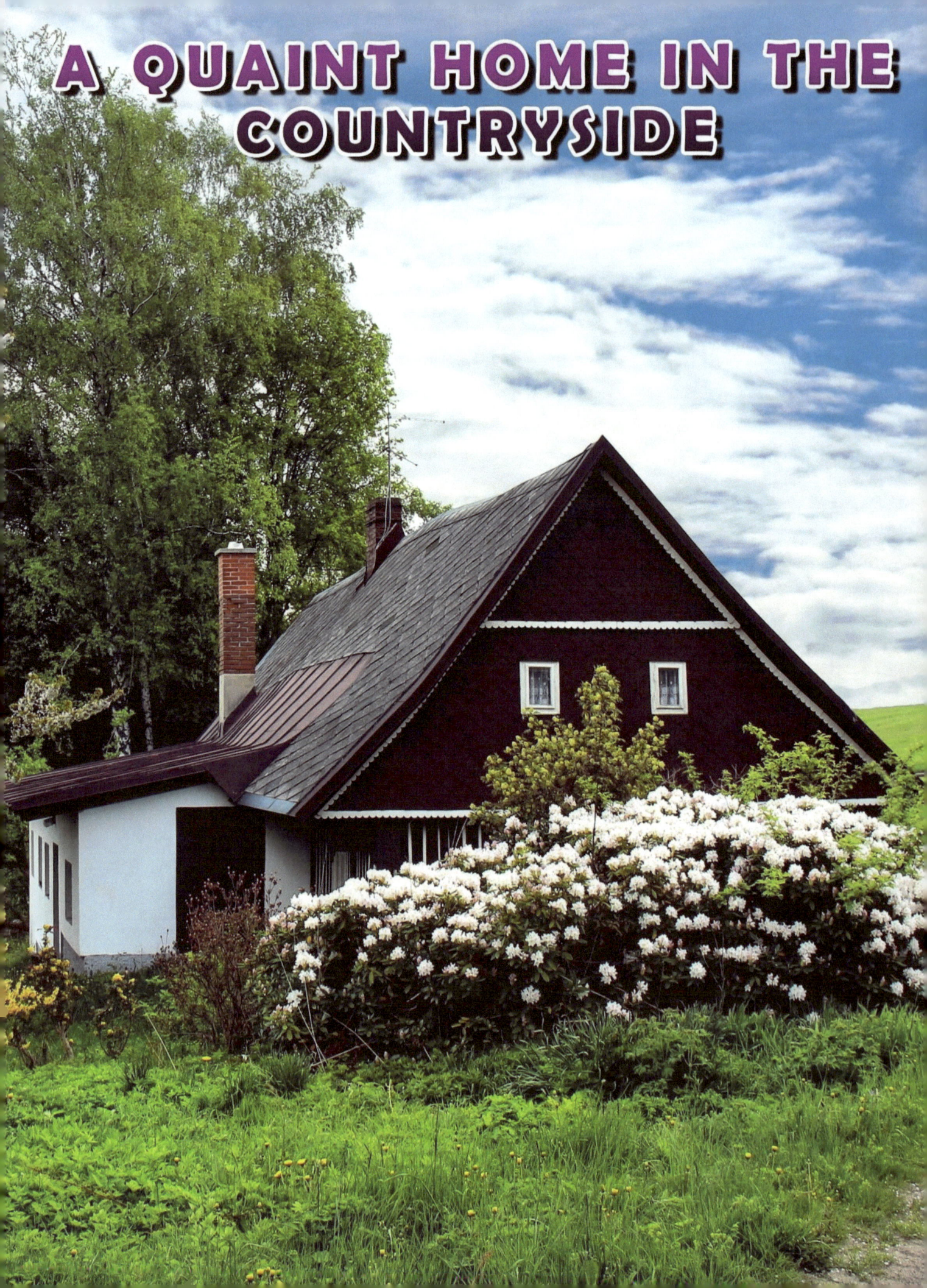

A QUAINT HOME IN THE COUNTRYSIDE

THE MAJESTIC PEACOCK

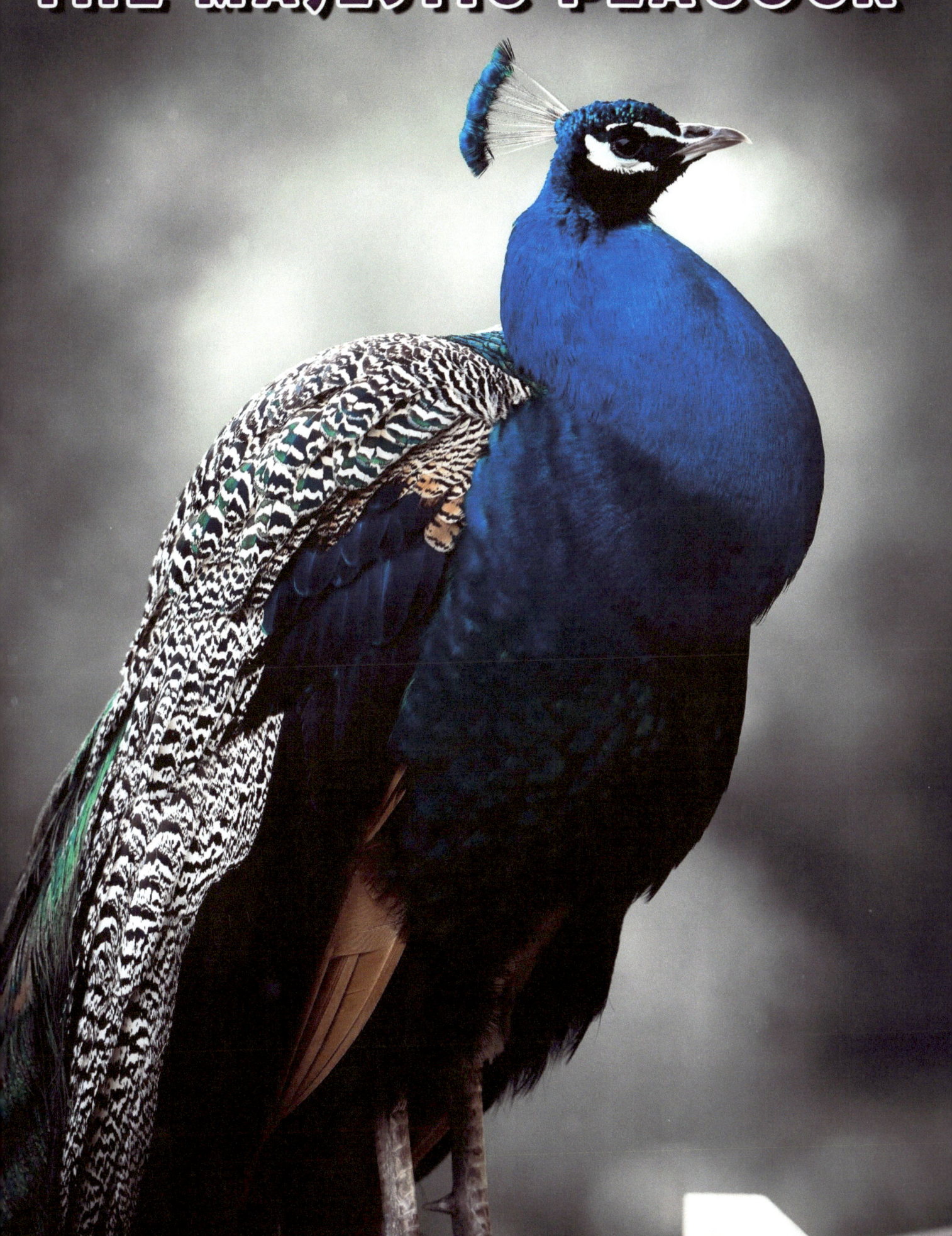

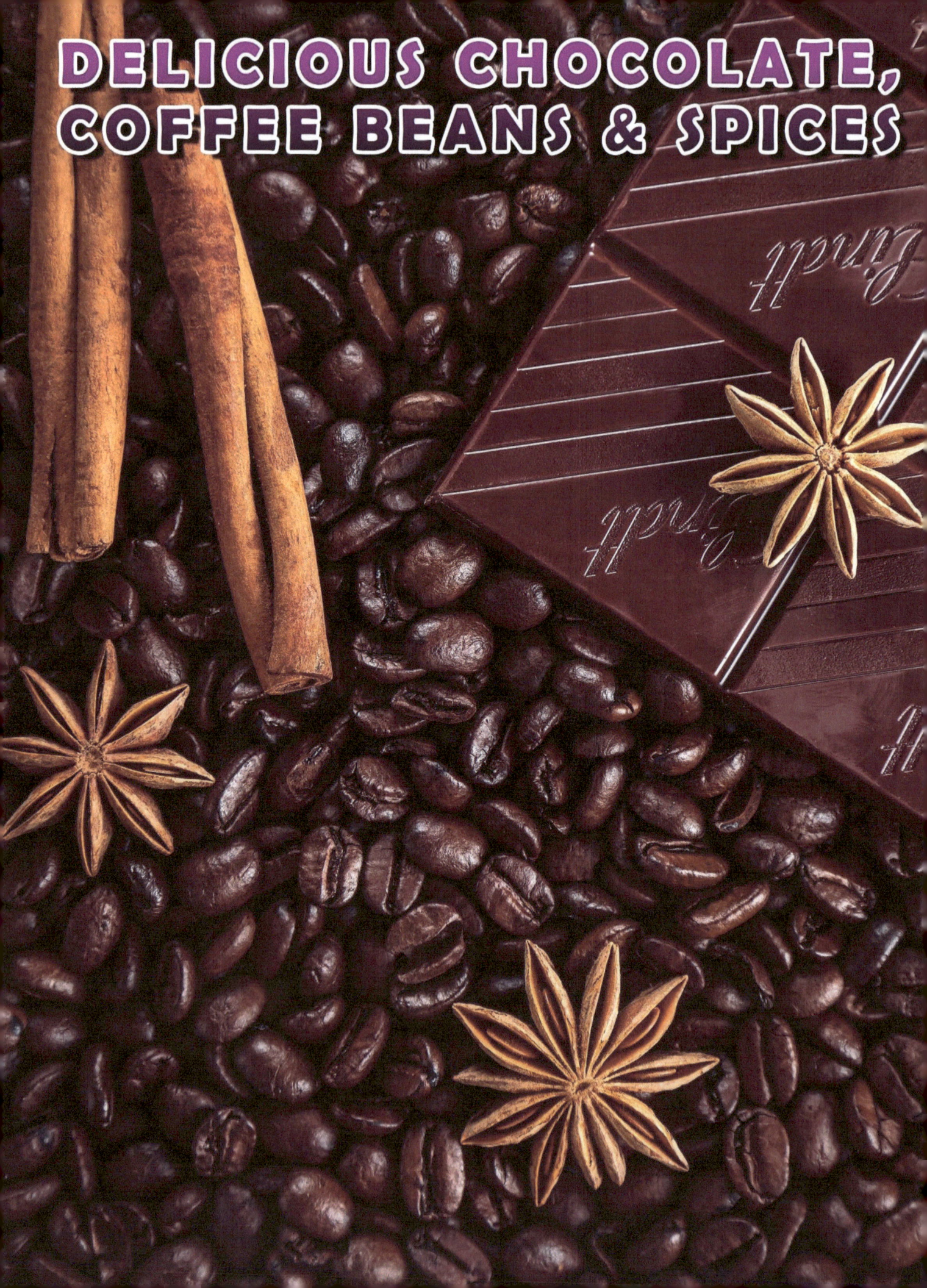

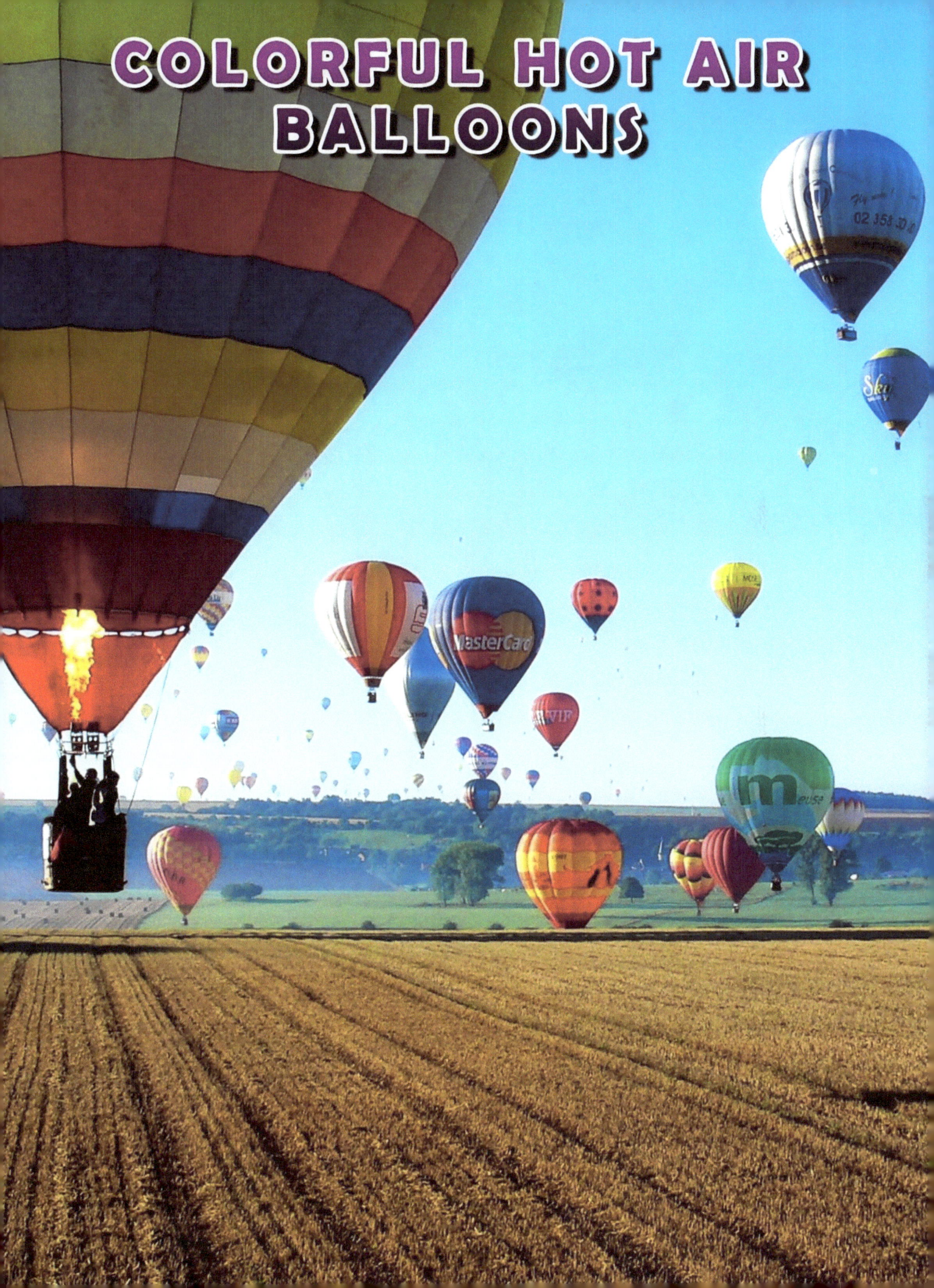

COLORFUL HOT AIR BALLOONS

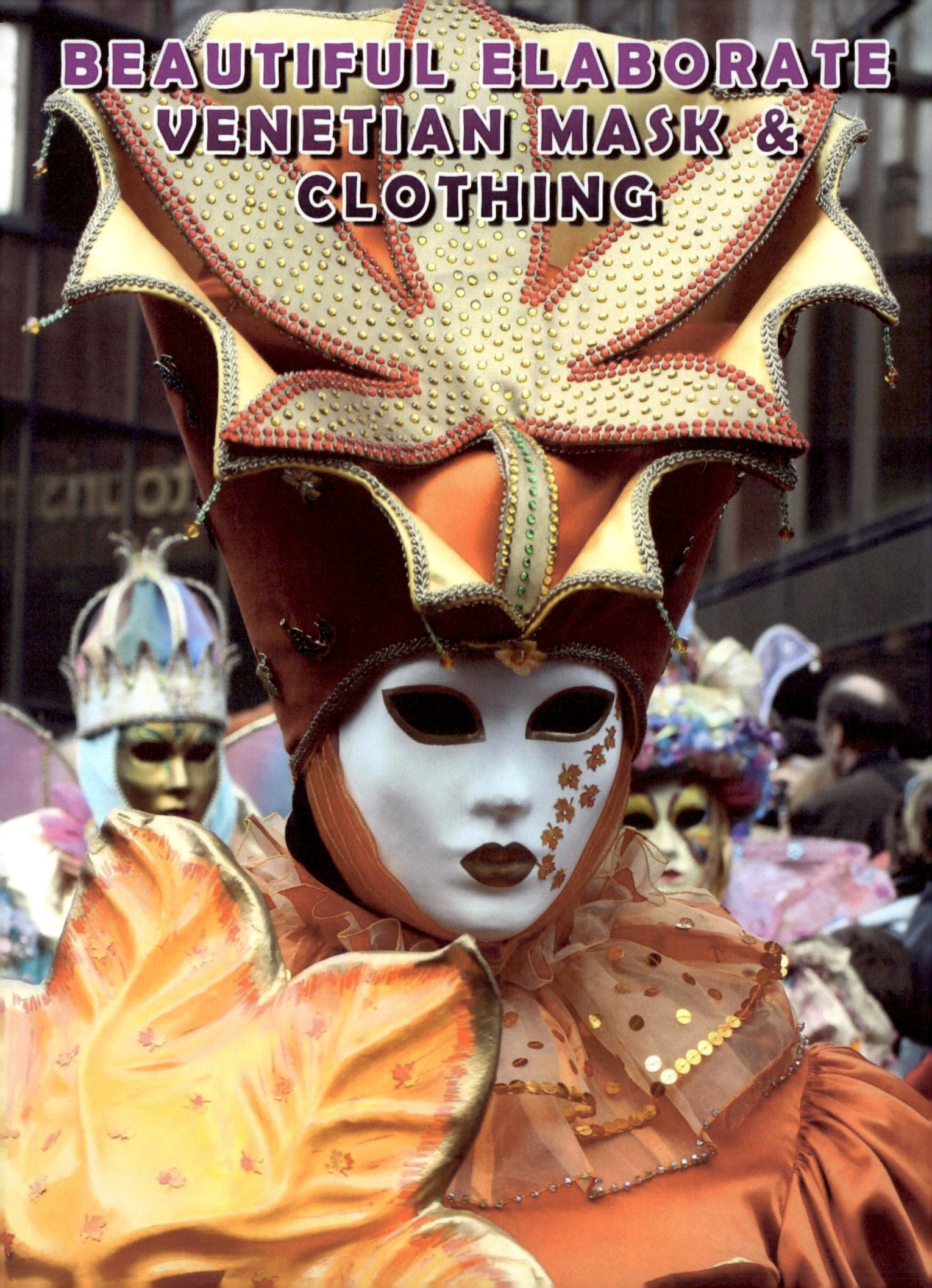

BEAUTIFUL ELABORATE VENETIAN MASK & CLOTHING

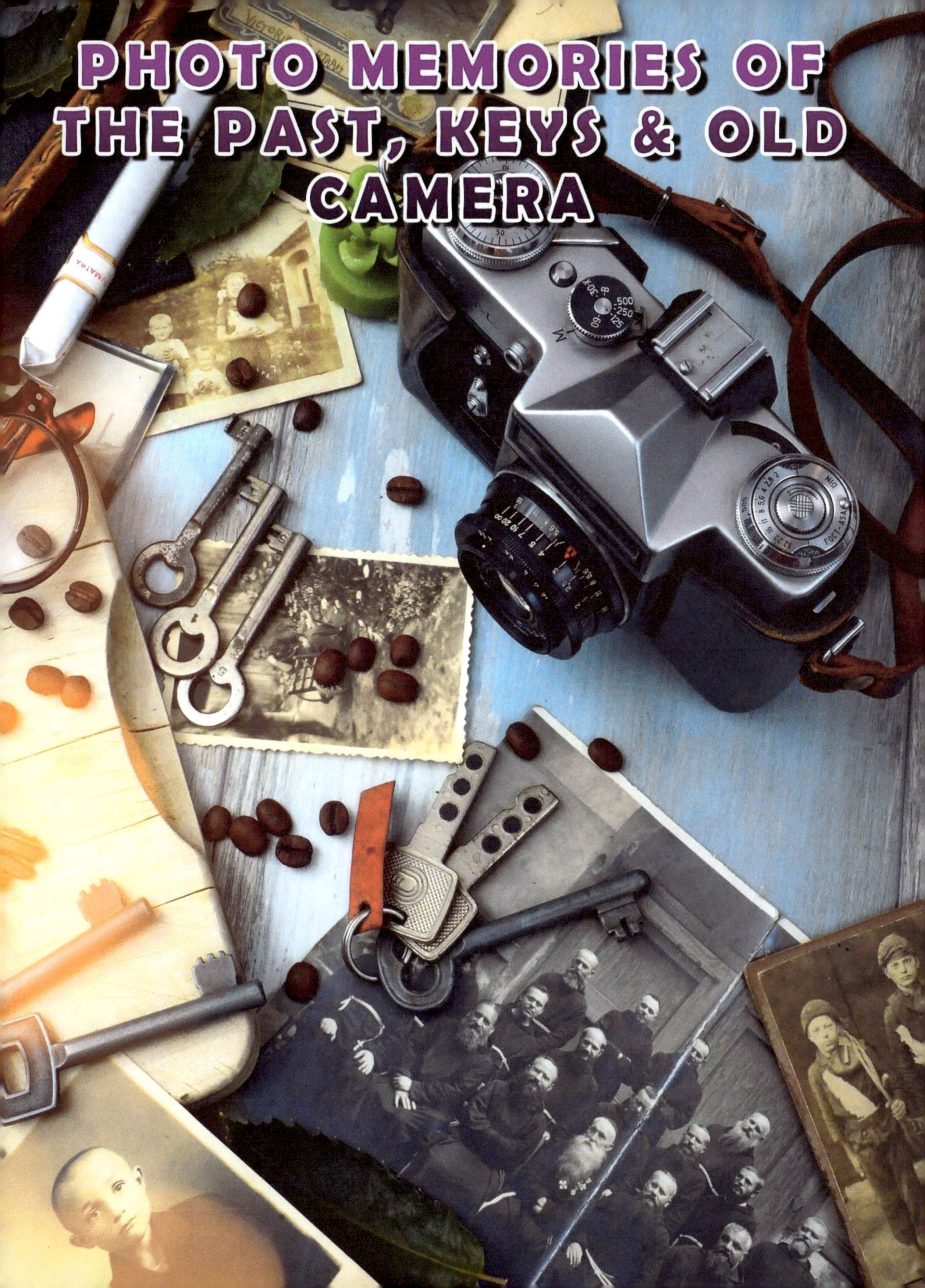

PHOTO MEMORIES OF THE PAST, KEYS & OLD CAMERA

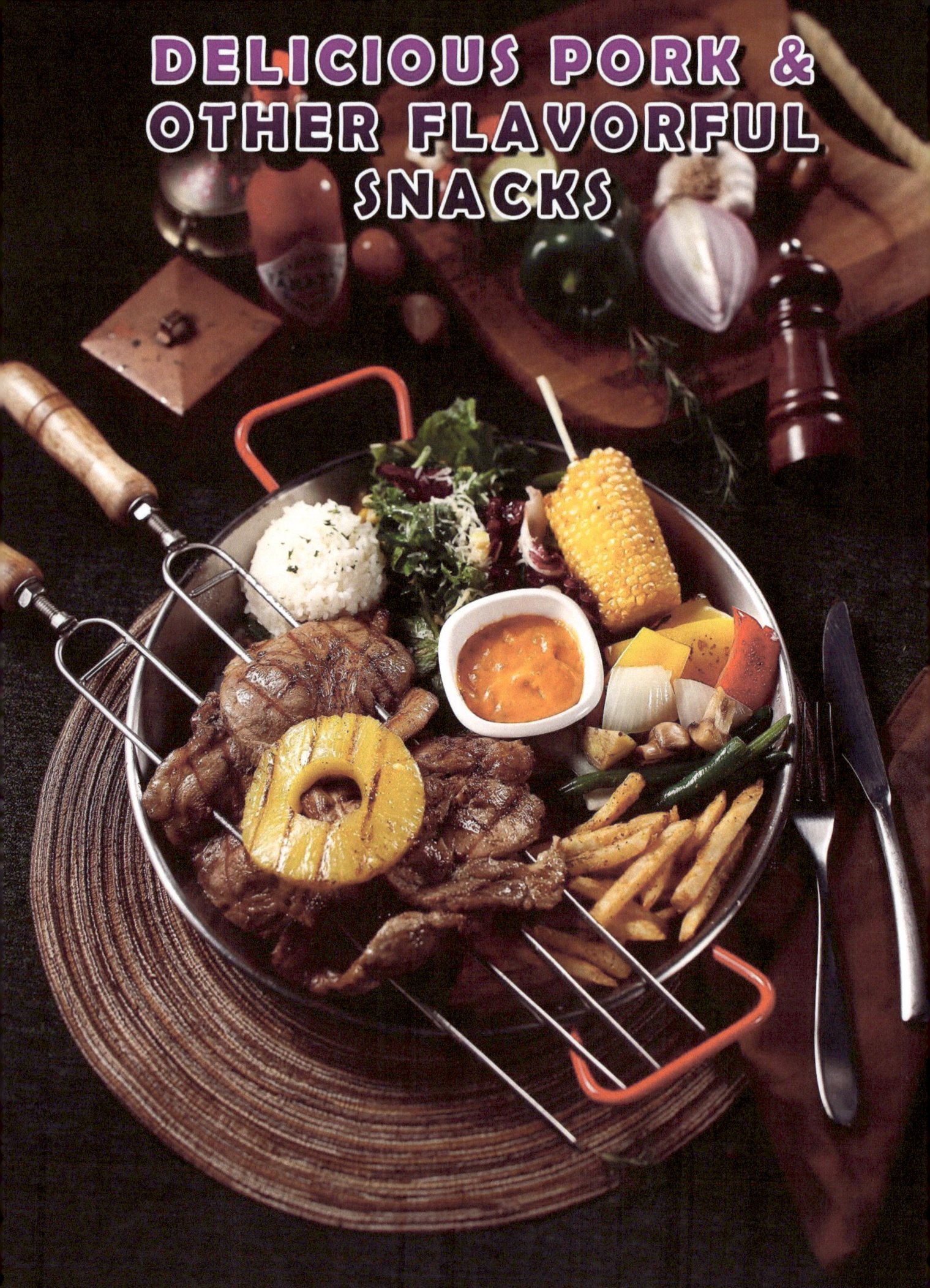

DELICIOUS PORK & OTHER FLAVORFUL SNACKS

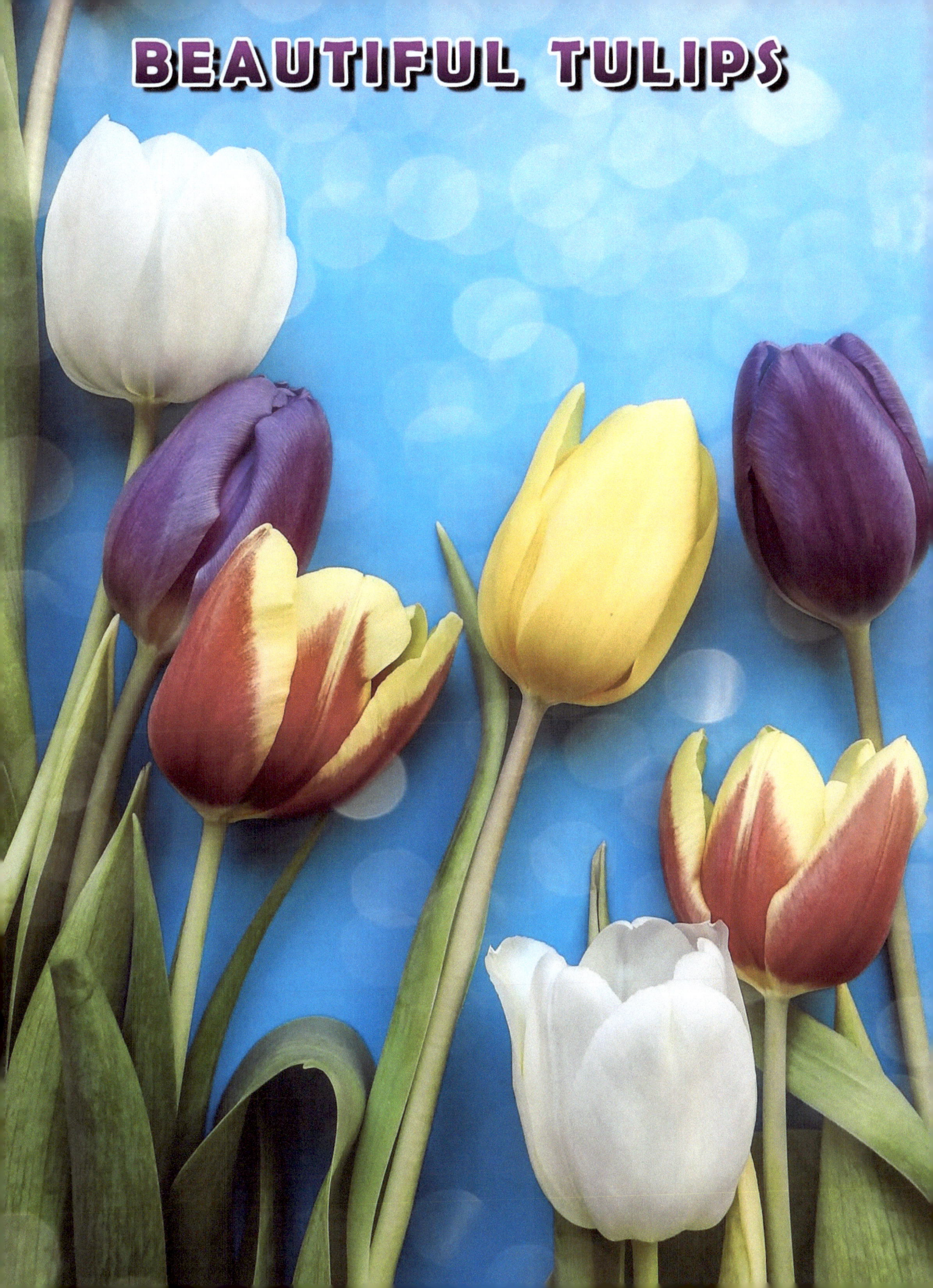

BEAUTIFUL TULIPS

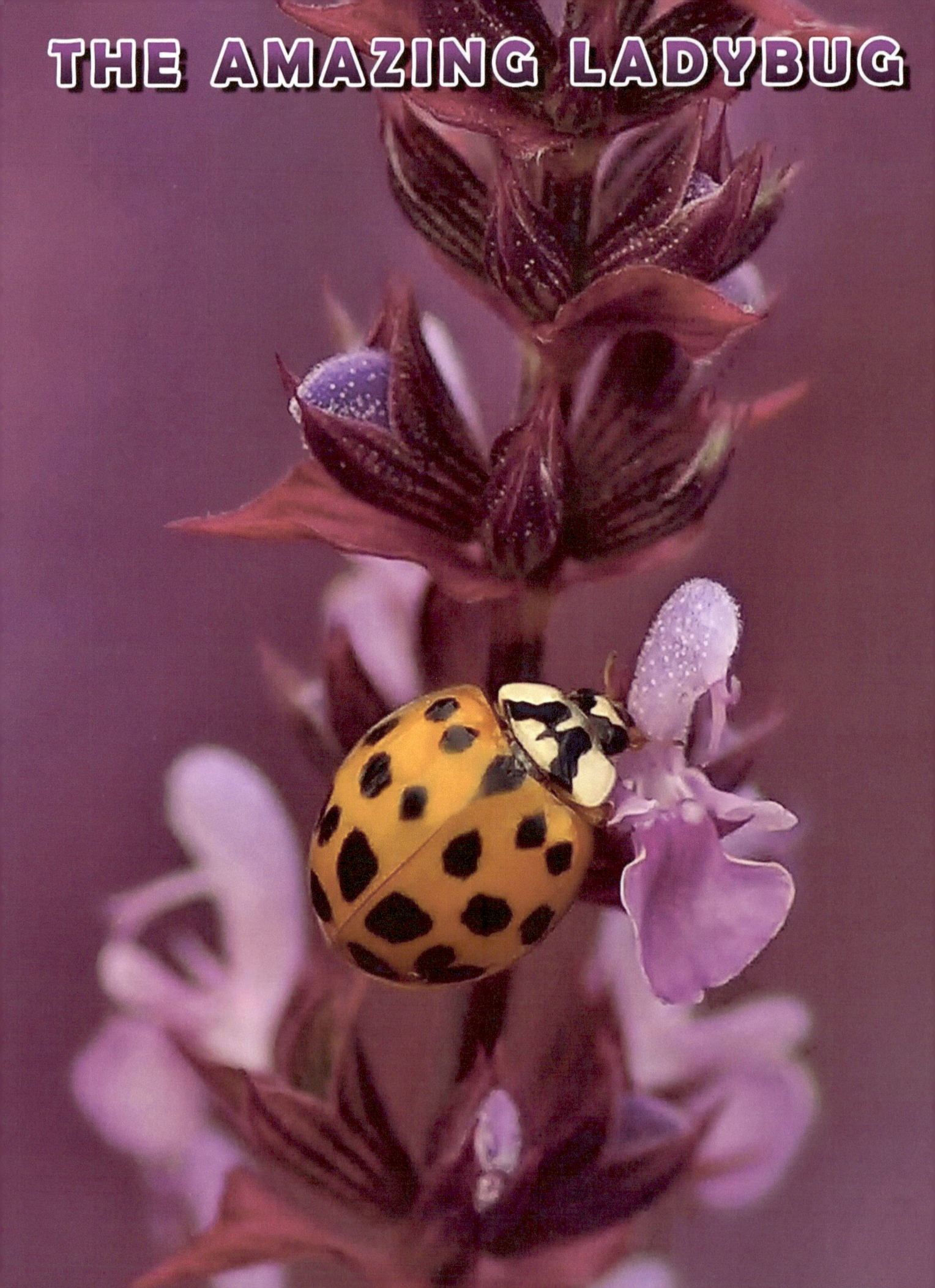

THE AMAZING LADYBUG

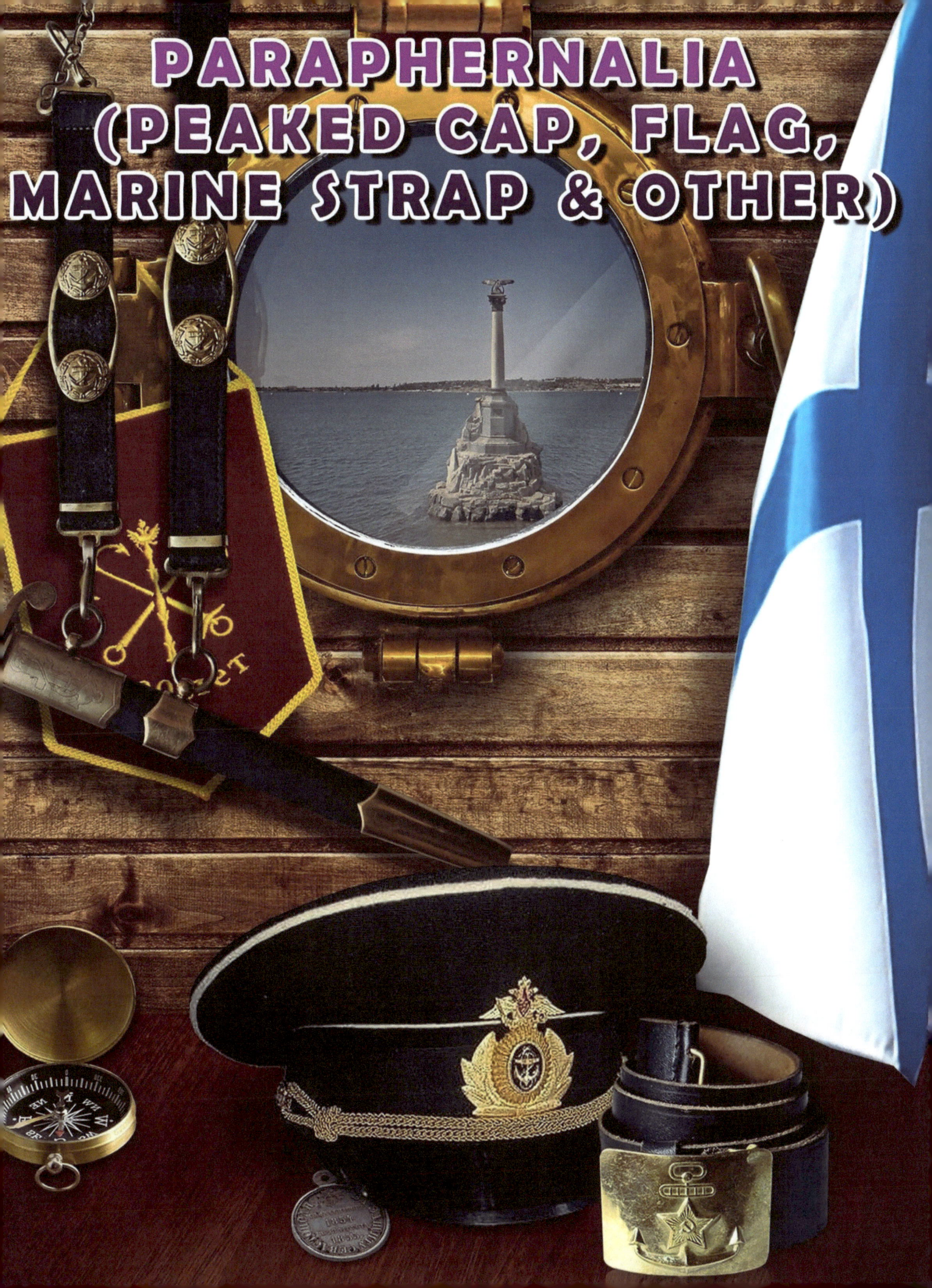

PARAPHERNALIA (PEAKED CAP, FLAG, MARINE STRAP & OTHER)

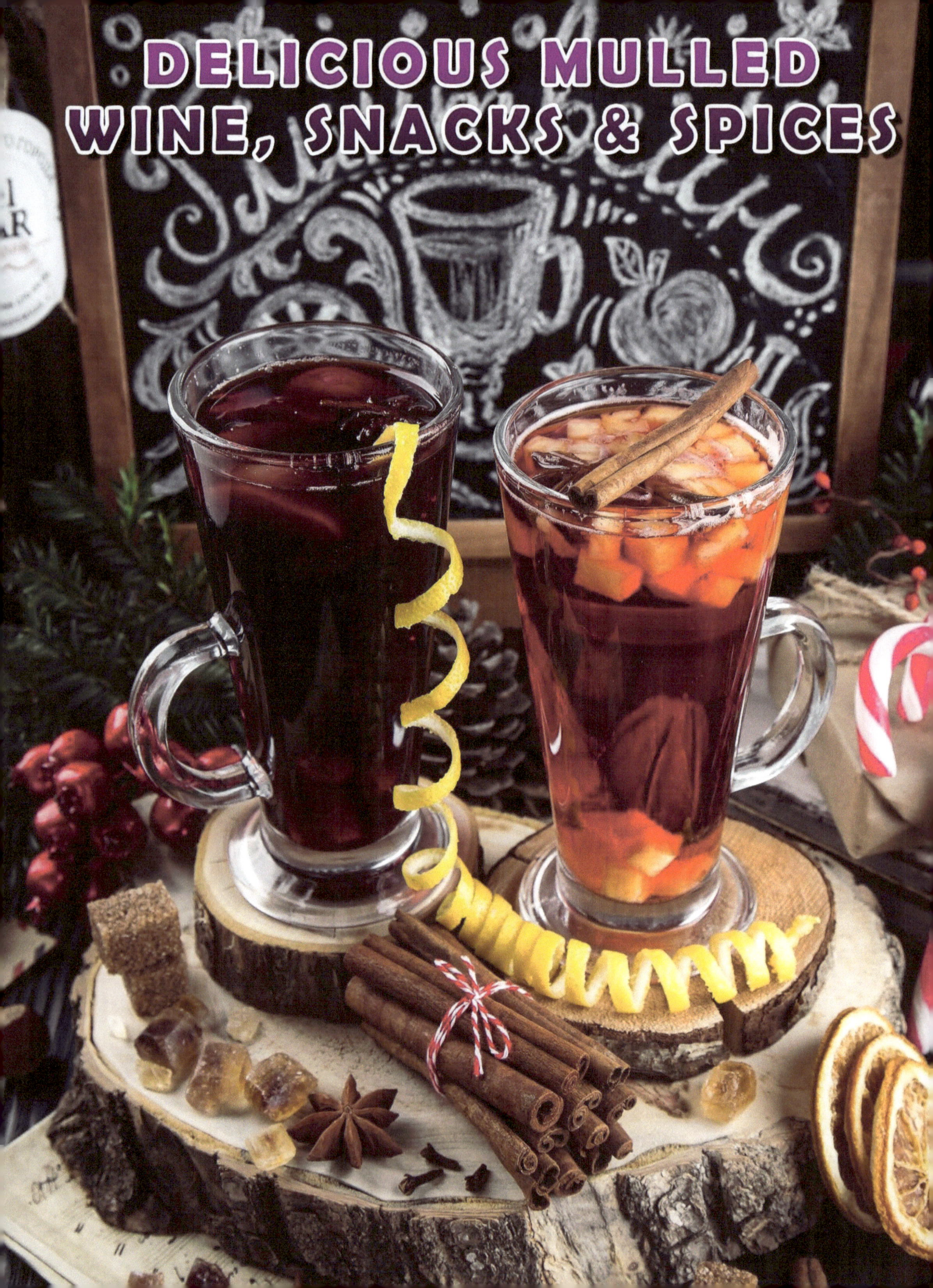

DELICIOUS MULLED WINE, SNACKS & SPICES

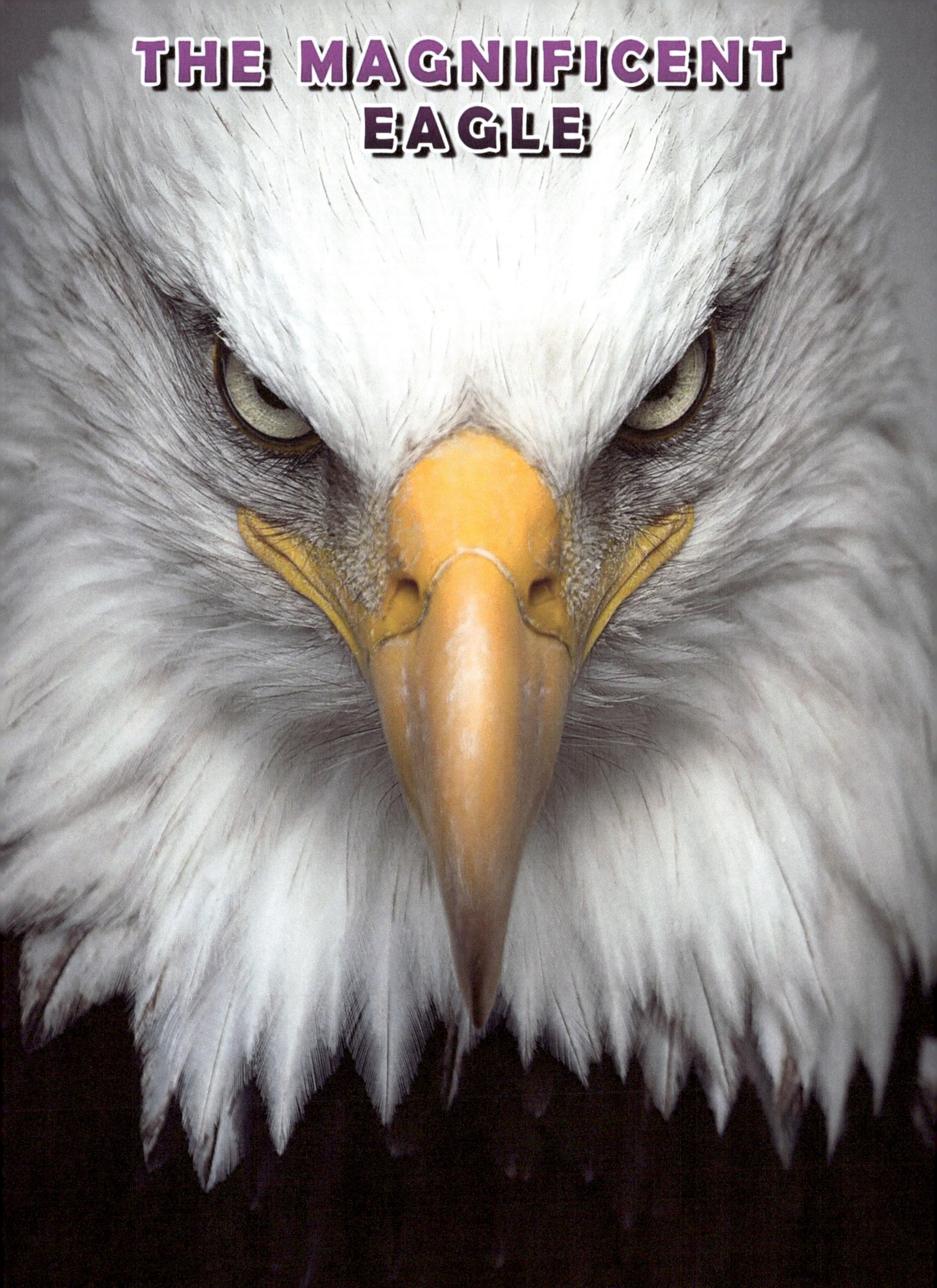

THE MAGNIFICENT
EAGLE

MILK COCKTAIL, VASE WITH FLOWERS & CAROUSEL ORNAMENT

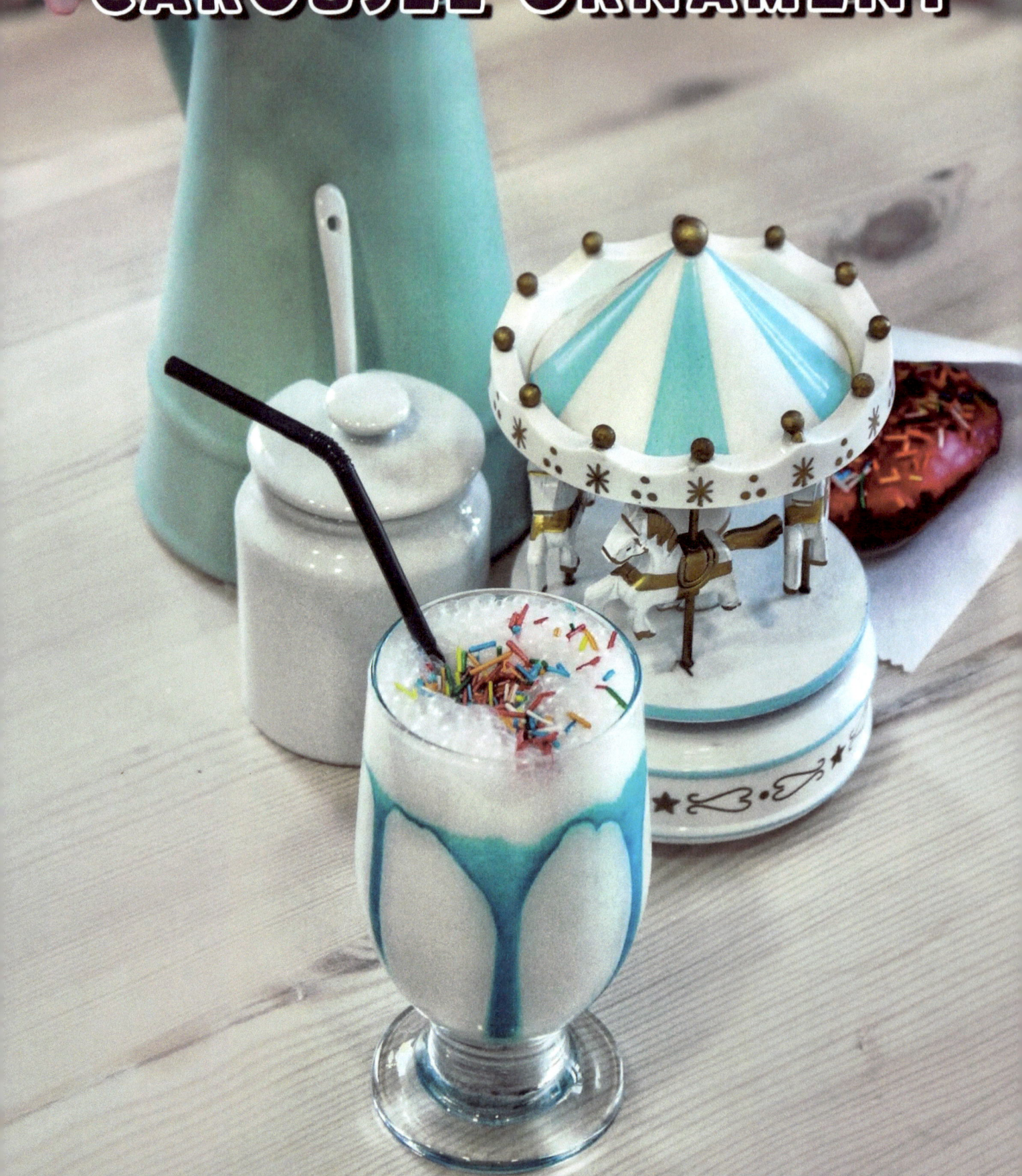

BIRDS PERCHED ON A BRANCH

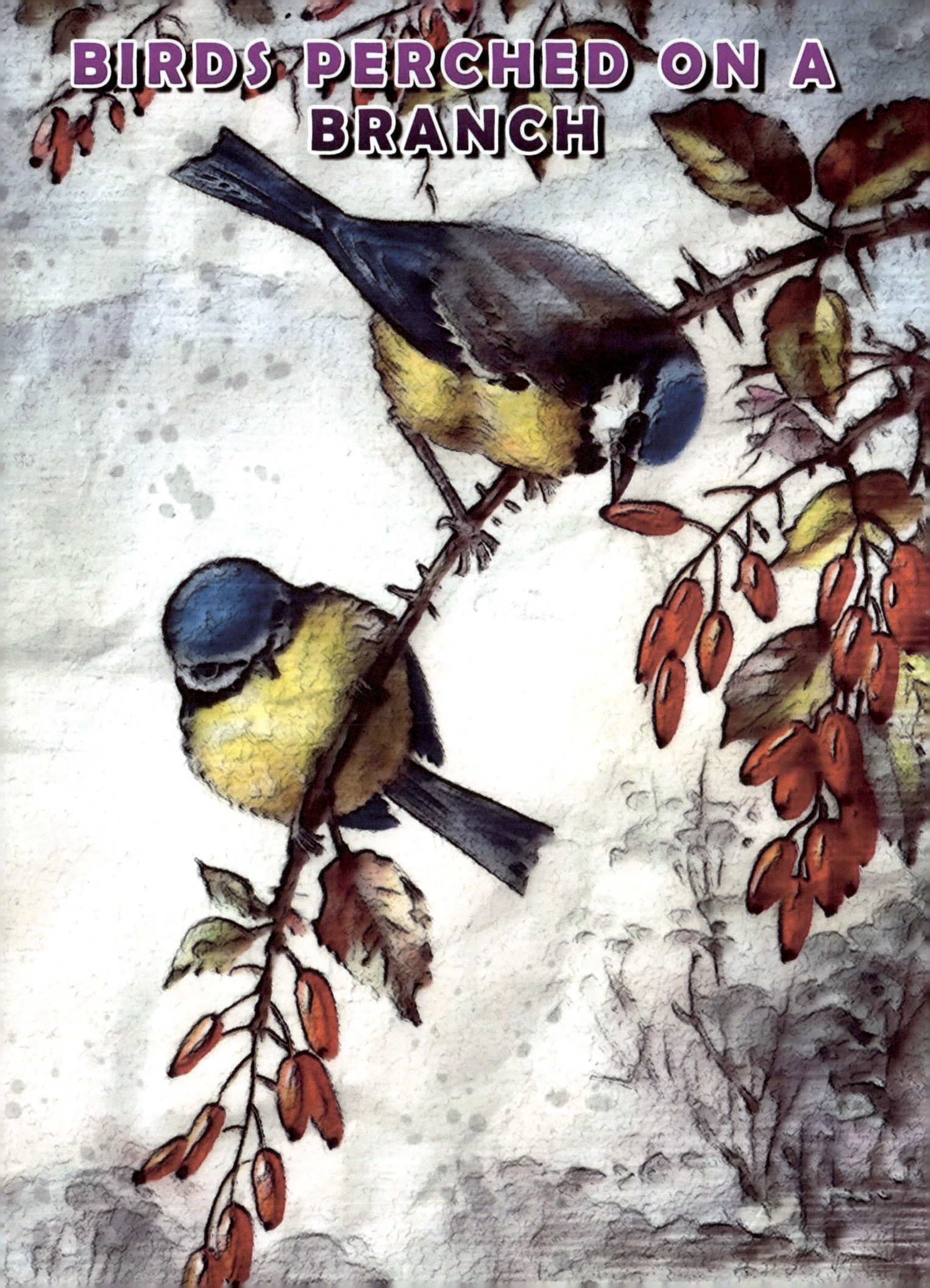

FANTASTIC

PICTURE BOOK: VARIOUS PICTURES

40 FULL COLOR IMAGES